Reproductive Efficiency of Female Cattle in the Tropic

Luis Orlando Alba Gómez, PhD
Full Professor and Consulting Professor
Discipline: Reproduction and Genetics

Notice

This is a complementary book that is intended to advise and guide those people who deal with the reproductive problems of female cattle. No two patients are the same. Therefore, we cannot be responsible for the actions or treatments administered to animals on farms without our supervision.

Reproductive Efficiency of Female Cattle in the Tropic

Copyright 2024 by Luis Orlando Alba Gomez
Cover Designer: Igor Alba Espinosa
Style review: Igor Alba Espinosa

All rights reserved

No part of this publication may be reproduced or transmited in any form or by any means, electronic or mechanical, without the written permission of the publisher.

Printer in the United States of America
Edited by Amazon Kindle Direct Publishing

Dedication

To my children and all those who collaborated in one way or another in the completion of this works

Acknowledgments

The many graduate students whom I scientifically guided in serious scientific-student activities, such as Coursework, Diploma Projects or in postgraduate activities such as Specialization and Doctoral Theses, deserve my particular recognition. The list of graduates would be too long to reproduce here, but many of their names appear in the references at the end of each chapter.

Preface

This work serves the purpose of providing students of Veterinary Medicine, Zootechnics, technicians, livestock farmers and professionals in the field, a useful source of information in which they can find reflected the most common problems that they face daily in the field of work. reproductive of the bovine female.

In its preparation I tried to ensure that the contents had to do with the most pressing reproductive problems of current tropical livestock farming and that is why it is not a very extensive book. Its main virtues are the innovative research results that are included and discussed and the agroecological and zootechnical approaches that are proposed to provide solutions to reproductive problems, along with the epizootiological work method that is required, to improve the reproductive efficiency of herds. in the tropics.

My intention is to educate the greatest possible number of professionals and practitioners in this field of Biology and to offer with this book an auxiliary means of training for individuals with diverse backgrounds, knowledge, and aspirations.

Index

Preface		1
Chap. 1	Gynecological work and its problems	3
Chap. 2	Regulation of reproductive functions	19
Chap. 3	Evaluation of reproductive performance	47
Chap. 4	Comparative genital anatomy	61
Chap. 5	Dysfunctions of the estrous cycle	94
Chap. 6	Inflammatory processes of the genital tract	113
Chap. 7	Abortion and its causes	137
Chap. 8	Congenital anomalies	149
Bibliography		157
Glossary		166
Biographical summary		168

Chapter 1

Gynecological work and its problems

Content:
Importance of the work method to use. Differences between the epizootiological and clinical methods. Strategy to carry out a comprehensive reproductive study of a herd. Clinical examination of the reproductive system.

Introduction

Despite the importance of bovine reproduction, there are few veterinarians and zootechnicians who serve this area effectively on farms or livestock companies. Perhaps the main reason is that they are not specialists, although there are others that have to do with personal preferences, aptitudes, and the inadequate conditions to carry out gynecological work in the dairy farms. All of this has the consequences that the fields of action of reproduction and zootechnics, which are within the functions of this profession, are only partially fulfilled. This chapter discusses possible ways to solve this problem.

Importance of the work method to use

There is a distinction between an emotional animal and a productive animal. The first can be provided with all the veterinary services requested by its owner, regardless of the costs. In the affectionate animal, it is justified to use the clinical method, appropriate for individual animals.

On the other hand, in productive animals economic and utilitarian considerations must prevail; then the most appropriate method of action is the epizootiological one.

For a better understanding of this matter, let's look at the meaning of the term Epizootiology and the concept of epizootiological method.

Epizootiology, in its narrowest sense, means the scientific study of epizootics, that is, it covers the problems that are related to the biological etiological agents that produce an infectious process, from viruses to protozoa and helminths.

Used in a broader sense, *Epizootiology* deals with the phenomena of animal health and morbidity related to all mass diseases, that is, it also studies the problems that are related to the agents and etiological factors that produce non-communicable diseases, for example, zoohygienic, reproductive, technology, management (*production diseases*) and diseases transmissible by inheritance. In addition, those caused by toxins, trauma, and dietary deficiencies.

Epizootiology deals not only with the epizootic processes of mass diseases but also with the collective health processes of herds and animal populations.

In this sense I want to highlight the epizootiological concept of animal health and disease that, in our cattle farming, is neither understood nor acted upon when it comes to animal malnutrition.

Animal Health
Comprises a biological system of a dynamic and multifactorial process in which animals are free of undesirable morphological or physiological deviations, as well as etiological agents that threaten the health of other animals or man, in such a way that, this process enables the use of animals and their products at a minimum level corresponding (*standardized*) to the species, breed and category determined in the given living conditions.

Animal Disease
Comprises the biological system of a dynamic and multifactorial process, in which animals are not free from undesirable morphological or physiological deviations or from etiological agents that threaten the health of other animals or man, so that this process reduces or makes impossible the use of these animals or their products, at least, to the level corresponding (*standardized*) to the species, breed and category, determined in the given living conditions.

The *nutritional status* of the animal population is one of the most important factors for collective health and mass diseases of animals, above all for resistance against diseases. Many flocks suffer from poor quantitative and qualitative nutrition during the drought period. However, this state of malnutrition, sometimes advanced, is not usually recognized as a nutritional disease. It then happens that entire herds suffering from malnutrition are milked and handled as if they were healthy animals.

Differences between the epizootiological and clinical methods

The *epizootiological method* has as its objects of study the populations and herds of animals, ecological agents and factors, sources, and routes of transmission and the environment. The health status is assessed considering healthy, suspicious, and affected animals. The research location is the animal breeding and production units. The time spent is medium and long term, continuous and systematic. Studies the epizootic and collective health process.

The *epizootiological diagnosis* is based on the impact of the herd or animal population by etiological or environmental agents. It proposes and establishes active, complete, extensive, programmed, systematic and operational preventive and recovery measures. The goals are outlined: to create, protect and recover the health of the herd or animal population, including the production of food in quantity and quality.

The *clinical method* has individual animals as its objects of study. The state of health is assessed from clinically sick animals. The place to investigate them is the place where the animal lives. The time spent is short-term, momentary, occasional. It establishes preventive and curative measures only for sick individuals who, due to their nature, are passive, occasional, and partial. The goal is to cure the sick animal, so the social, health, economic and productive effectiveness is very limited. It does not intervene in food production or ecological problems.

According to the above, to diagnose and favorably resolve reproductive problems, which in cattle farming are multifactorial, it is necessary to use the epizootiological method and consider the herd as the object. The clinical method will be used only as a complementary method to help specify the diagnosis in the herd.

Strategy for the comprehensive reproductive study of a herd

As is already known, the reproductive efficiency of an individual depends on the homeostasis of its internal environment. This balance can be broken by the harmful action of some factors. Therefore, the best strategy to follow is to study them by actions, in an orderly manner.

The first action consists of personally studying the microclimate in which the animals live. To do this, the grassland area must be inspected, type, quality, degree of infestation of undesirable plants, etc. Verify the presence or absence of forage areas and protein banks for nutritional assurance. Existence of natural or artificial shade areas to avoid heat stress. Presence or not of trees in the pastures and fences. Quantity and location of watering holes. Write down the findings in a notebook to establish an improvement plan.

The second action is the external inspection of pregnant and empty cows and heifers, to judge their nutritional status. To do this, special attention will be paid to the protruding needles of the dorsal vertebrae, ribs, prominences of the lumbar processes, iliac and ischial tuberosities, as well as the tail mass.

In castle females with a good state of nutrition, the different body regions appear well delimited; However, thick adipose panicles can still be seen. In those of fair condition or skinny, the body surfaces are flattened, highlighting the muscular contours; There is no adipose panniculus, but neither does any part of the skeleton stand out intensely; the skin remains elastic.

In castle females with *a poor state of nutrition*, the bone parts already mentioned are very evident and the skin is intensely adhered to the skeleton.

These states of primary undernutrition are generally accompanied by symptoms of anemia such as paleness of the visible mucous membranes, edema of the submandibular skin and physical changes in the blood, which becomes light red in color and not very viscous (fluid).

A simple way to detect anemia clinically is by inspection of the episcleral vessels. For the examination, the animal's head is twisted to one side, which rotates the eyeball and exposes it.

The fullness, limits and coloring must be considered, as well as the possible pulsation of these glasses. In bovines they appear moderately full and well manifested, that is, standing out from the immediate parts. Empty episcleral vessels, which poorly define their contours, are symptoms of overt anemia.

The third action is to carry out a study of the reproductive status of the herd and, in addition, obtain the individual and collective reproductive indices, as explained in Chapter 3.

After the data have been analyzed and a presumptive diagnosis has been reached, a random selection of 10-15 % of the affected cows will be made to be gynecologically explored, if the herd is 100-120 cows, if is 50, select 10 and if it is 25, seven or eight.

The **fourth action** is to carry out the gynecological diagnosis of the selected females, to reach the definitive diagnosis. An individual record of the clinical findings observed should be kept.

The **fifth action** is to propose and establish active, programmed, systematic and operational preventive and recovery measures in the short, medium, and long term, with the purpose of making the necessary adjustments and protecting and recovering the health of the herd, including the production of food in quantity and in quality.

How to get started in the gynecological work of a flock

Of the five basic actions already mentioned, the fourth action, which is the gynecological study of a percentage of the herd, is important, but not essential, since it is done to confirm a presumptive diagnosis of the reproductive status of the herd.

If the reality is accepted that more than 95% of the reproductive disorders that affect tropical livestock are environmental and zootechnical, the reproductive efficiency of the herd could be substantially improved, if the epizootiological method already proposed is used and the adjustments made are made. require, in a timely manner.

As an additional strategy, the Veterinarian-zootechnician, not a specialist in Gynecology, can be assisted by an inseminator technician or an average veterinary technician with experience in rectal examination, to carry out pregnancy diagnoses and verify the presence or absence of CLs. in the ovaries in cases of functional anestrus or acquire and use a portable ultrasound machine. (See Chapter 4).

Clinical examination of the reproductive system

Transrectal palpation

Palpation of the internal genitalia through the rectal wall continues to be one of the most valuable tools used in reproductive management programs in cattle, since it provides all the necessary information, in addition to being very fast, practical, and economical.

The clothing required is overalls or overalls, high rubber boots and optionally a rubber apron or apron.

The minimum equipment consists of disposable nylon obstetric gloves, which cover the professional's hand and arm to protect them from direct contact with the female's fecal matter; a leaflet speculum for heifers and another for cows, a flashlight or light source for vaginoscopy, a Janet or other 100 cm^3 plastic syringe, semi-rigid plastic or rubber catheters, antiseptics, and soap.

Additionally, a clipboard with paper to record the clinical findings observed.

Fixation procedures for exploration

Some dairy cows, especially those of European breeds, are docile and have little tendency to kick. The transrectal examination can be performed on them without taking them to the stocks. However, crossbred females and zebu with little contact with humans are irritable and kick when you try to explore them.

For this reason, they must be placed in a trap to fix them and be able to work safely. This is important to ensure the physical protection of the operator. Furthermore, when working with fear, diagnostic skills are greatly reduced.

Transrectal exploration technique and its effectiveness

How to perform transrectal examination is taught in undergraduate Gynecology practical classes and the theoretical aspects are described in Animal Reproduction textbooks. However, the practical classes received in the undergraduate degree are not enough for students to acquire the necessary skills. For this reason, the professional who wishes to specialize in Vaccine Gynecology must do so on their own. I note that all the authors of Veterinary Gynecology textbooks that I know tend to simplify the explanations of the diagnostic possibilities of rectal palpation. Others exaggerate them.

In this part I will try to give its fair value to the diagnostic effectiveness of transrectal exploration, according to my personal experience.

The gloved hand should be wet with water to act as a lubricant. To overcome the resistance of the anal sphincter, you must first introduce one finger, then two, three and finally close your hand in a cone shape and penetrate forcefully, moving your hand. If the defecation reflex is stimulated, hand movement should be suspended during the peristaltic wave.

If fecal matter is in the way of the examination, it should be removed so that only the rectal wall remains between the hand and the reproductive system. This must be done without removing the hand from the rectum, otherwise air penetrates, and peristalsis is suspended. This causes the rectal blister to distend as if it were a board, making palpation impossible.

To perform rectal palpation correctly, the same exploratory routine must be followed. The pelvic cavity is first inspected to locate and fix the cervix by hand. This maneuver is essential since its fixation allows palpation of the rest of the genital apparatus. If the organ is not located in that location, the hand should move deeper into the abdominal cavity, somewhat in front of the anterior edge of the pubis.

The second step is to fix the uterus tightly by the intercornual ligament and retract it into the pelvic cavity so that the uterus can be examined more easily. If the uterus is heavy and not retractable, there is a probability that the female is pregnant for 4 or more months.

Once the retraction has been carried out, the cervix is examined for size, shape, and consistency. Next, the horns are palpated for size, wall thickness, content and especially tone, which is the sign that best predicts the ovarian hormonal status in real time.

Relaxed and flaccid uterine horns correspond to inactive ovaries or in the diestral phase. The horns that harden slightly when palpated correspond to ovaries that have some degree of estrogenic activity.

The size, thickness of the uterine wall and content are important elements for gynecological diagnosis; but its tactile interpretation has a high degree of difficulty because the uterus changes depending on the phase of the sexual cycle in which the female is.

Uterine palpation allows effective diagnosis of pregnancy in quite early stages, serves to verify the postpartum involution process, recognize structural changes during the estrous cycle and detect some anatomical abnormalities. However, it does not allow us to specify the diagnosis of chronic endometritis.

Palpation of the fallopian tubes is almost impracticable due to the extreme thinness of the oviduct and the softness of the tubal ampulla and infundibulum that makes them almost unrecognizable through the rectal wall.

This extraordinary thinness of the oviducts and the tightness of the closure of the uterine-tubal junction constitute an insurmountable barrier to the passage of toxins, gases, liquids, and germs from the uterine contents. Perhaps this is why inflammatory disorders of the fallopian tubes are so rare in female cattle.

The last step is the examination of the ovaries. To check them it is not necessary to retract them, it is enough to locate the broad ligament and locate the gonad by taking it in the palm and turning the hand in such a way that it is above the palm and the ovarian ligament, between the ring and middle fingers, leaving the thumb and index finger, which are passed over the ovarian surface to determine its size, shape and consistency. For beginners, locating and fixing the ovaries, mainly the left one, is extremely difficult.

A distinction must be made between locating and fixing the internal genital organs and knowing how to recognize and interpret what is palpated. To learn the first, it is necessary to perform rectal palpation on many animals frequently and systematically, until the technique is mastered.

To interpret, through touch, what is palpated, extensive theoretical knowledge of Anatomy and Reproductive Pathophysiology is required and, in addition, exercise using the technique of tactile memory.

The word tactile means: having qualities perceptible by touch, or that suggest such perception. Tactile memory consists of identifying and mentally representing the qualities of an organ that is palpated. It is acquired by dissecting the genital organs of heifers and cows in different phases of the estrous cycle. For example, take an ovary, observe it carefully to see its shape, if it has follicles or CL, that is, study its macroscopic structure. Then measure it with a caliper to find out its size in centimeters. Finally, take the ovary between your fingers and without looking at it, palpate it gently with your fingertips, repeatedly to recognize its consistency and to remember what you measured, saw and felt.

The presence of small tertiary follicles can be deduced (not palpated) by the elastic or slightly fluctuating consistency of the ovaries. A completely inactive gonad has a hard-elastic, or more compact, consistency. Tertiary follicles larger than seven mm are palpable as light pockets that stand out on the surface of the ovary.

Preovulatory follicles reach a diameter of 1.5 to 2 cm and are palpable as soft, fluctuating prominences on their surface.

The mature or Graafian follicle cannot be palpated because it forms a few hours before ovulation.

The CL can be safely palpated when it is well developed, starting 10 to 12 days into the cycle. It is recognized by the change in shape of the gonad, by a slight bulge that protrudes from the surface of the ovary and by the different consistency of the ovarian environment with respect to the CL. Sometimes, a CL of 2.5-3.0 cm in diameter is very included within the ovary and does not make any prominence.

Recognition of the CL by palpation is very important for the diagnosis of pregnancy and functional anestrus, since its presence means that ovulation has occurred, and the animal is in the progesterone phase.

A cow with repeat breeding may contain, in its ovaries, several CLs in different involutional phases. During involution, the prominence becomes smaller and smaller, until it almost disappears. A CL in the corpus rubrum phase is impalpable. The corpus albicans much less so.

Ovarian tumors in cattle occur very rarely and are recognized clinically by the significant increase in their volume and the hardness of their consistency.

A teratoma (*tumor composed of several types of tissues*) is palpated as a compact mass with an irregular surface, covering the entire gonad. It can reach the size of a chicken egg or more. Granulosa cell tumors can reach the size of a large round melon and weigh about 15 kg (Fig. 1-1). Due to its large size, this ovarian tumor is impalpable, and its discovery is almost always postmortem.

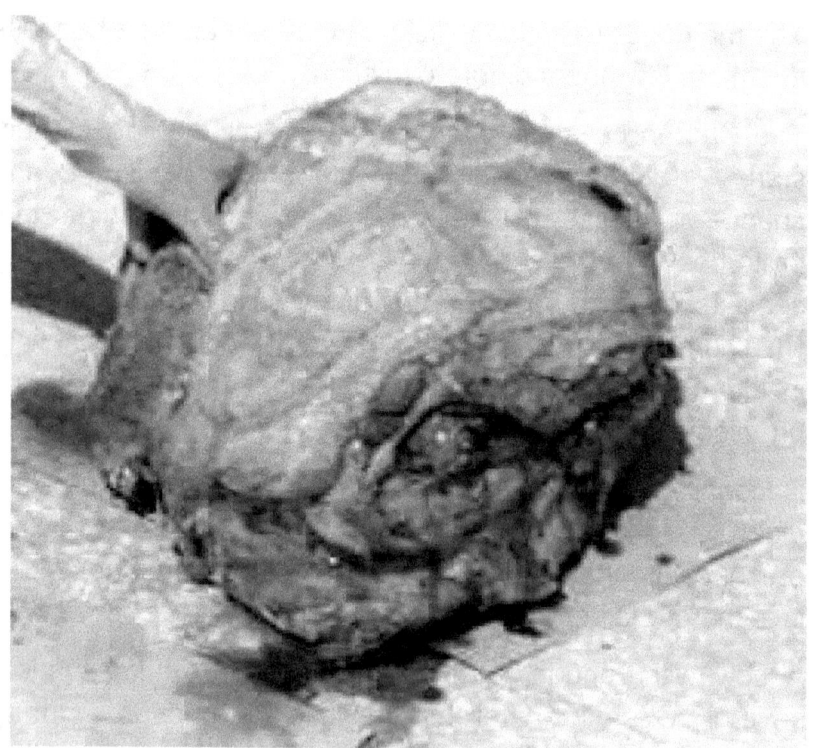

Fig. 1-1 Ovarian tumor

The value of the theoretical description of how gynecological processes and disorders in bovine females are diagnosed by touch is undoubted.

But this knowledge is assimilated much better by the clinician after having learned to palpate and exercise the technique of tactile memory, which is his best teacher.

Vaginal exploration

To perform vaginoscopy, you need to have two well-nickel-plated specula with leaflets, two plastic or metal buckets with a 10-liters capacity, an antiseptic to disinfect the water and the specula, and a light source.

It is important that there is enough drinking water at the examination site to adequately clean the vulva and anus.

Since vaginoscopy is a diagnostic adjunct, the transrectal examination should be performed first. This way you can completely empty the rectal ampoule and prevent the speculum from getting dirty during the examination. On the other hand, air entering the vagina can cause expulsive tenesmus and make rectal exploration difficult.

Before proceeding, both buckets are prepared with disinfected water and the specula are placed in each of them. That way, while one is used the other is disinfected. The speculum used is cleaned of remains of mucus and feces with plenty of drinking water and placed inside the bucket with disinfectant.

Once the external cleaning of the female has been carried out, the speculum is taken by its fixed handle and placed with its beak parallel to the entrance of the vulva. The resistance of the hymenal ring is overcome by pushing the instrument inward with moderate force.

It is important that the body of the speculum penetrates deeply, to be able to rotate and open the valves, without causing traumatic injuries to the vagina.

Indications for vaginoscopy

Due to the requirements, vaginal examination is not routinely used in gynecological examination; but it is a good complement to transrectal palpation, in some specific situations. For example, in the confirmatory diagnosis of chronic cervico-vaginitis and endometritis, which appears in Chapter. 6.

Chapter 2

Regulation of reproductive functions

Content:
Hypothalamic and neurohypophysis hormones. Ovarian hormones. Hormonal regulation mechanism of the sexual cycle. Therapeutic forms to use. Grouping of oestrus with intra-vaginal devices. PGF2α analogues. Induction of labor with PGF2α. Early diagnosis of non-pregnancy. Hormonal immunoneutralization. Immunization against PMSG.

Introduction

For the veterinarian who practices gynecology in cattle to achieve satisfactory results, he must master the basic physiological aspects of reproductive endocrinology and the neuro-hormonal processes involved in the mechanism of regulation of the estrous cycle.

Based on this knowledge, he will be able to better interpret and decide the type of exogenous hormone required.

Hypothalamic hormones

Two types of neurohormones are formed at the level of the hypothalamus.

a) Gonadotropin releasing hormone (GnRH)

GnRHs are decapeptides with a molecular weight of 1183 and are formed in the median eminence. Its function is to stimulate the secretion and release of the gonadotropic hormones FSH and LH, produced in the anterior lobe of the pituitary gland.

b) Neurohypophysis hormones

These are oxytocin and vasopressin. Both are formed in the supraoptic and paraventricular nuclei of the hypothalamus.

Oxytocin acts on the contractility of the smooth muscle fibers of the previously estrogenized uterus and on the myoepithelial cells of the udder related to milk ejection.

Vasopressin influences water reabsorption in the distal part of the renal tubules.

Actions of oxytocin in the estrous cycle

During heat, oxytocin discharges occur that activate the contractility of the uterus, which allows the seminal material to rise to the oviducts in a few minutes.

Oxytocin produced in the follicular area participates in the ovulation mechanism; The one produced in the corpus luteum at the end of diestrus stimulates the synthesis and secretion of $PGF2\alpha$ so that luteolysis occurs.

Pituitary gonadotropins

They are two hormones that are synthesized and accumulate in the anterior lobe of the pituitary gland. Its effector or target organ is the ovary.

Follicle stimulating hormone (FSH)

Chemically it is a water-soluble glycoprotein. Its main function is to stimulate the growth, development, and maturation of pre-cavitary follicles in the ovaries. In the presence of LH, it stimulates the production of ovarian estrogens.

Luteinizing hormone (LH)

It is a glycoprotein, and its biological activity is linked to the protein fraction. It acts synergistically with FSH, completes follicular maturation, activates the ovulating enzyme complex so that ovulation occurs and contributes to the formation and maintenance of the corpus luteum (CL).

Ovarian hormones

Estrogens

The estrogens produced in the ovaries are: 17β-estradiol and estron. Its synthesis is carried out by the granulosa cells of the theca interna of the De Graaf follicles, during heat.

Biological action

Estrogens ensure the development of female characteristics, the maturity of the genito-mammary apparatus and the regular succession of the estrous cycle.

The three morphological modifications that estrogen produces in the genital organs and especially on the uterus are: edema, hyperemia and cell growth (epithelial and muscle).

During the follicular phase, it produces an increase in blood supply to the genital organs and irritability of the myometrium. Furthermore, they condition the uterus and prepare it for the following progestative phase and reduce the threshold of excitability of the hypothalamic sexual center so that the psychic signs of heat are manifested.

On the other hand, estrogens influence bone growth by intensifying the development of the epiphyseal ends; They promote the retention of P, Na and Ca and stimulate the secretion of STH, which is used for fattening animals.

The effects of estrogens on the mammary gland differ depending on the reproductive state of the animal. In heifers, estrogens produce complete development of the epithelium of the milk canals and glandular acinis, that is, they are galacto-stimulators. On the contrary, in cows they are galacto-inhibitors, which is why during heat, milk production is slightly affected.

Progestogens

The main one is progesterone secreted by the CL and the placenta. Chemically it is a ketosteroid, an interproduct of corticosteroids and androgens. It does not accumulate in the body and has a very short biological half-life. It circulates through the blood along with plasma proteins, and is converted into pregnandiol in the liver, which is conjugated with glucuronic acid and is thus excreted through the urine.

Biological action

Progesterone (P_4) is essentially the hormone of gestation. During the sexual cycle, progesterone acts synergistically with estrogens, transforming the proliferative phase into the secretory phase. On the other hand, during pregnancy, P_4 antagonizes estrogen, inhibiting cervical secretion, uterine and fallopian tube motility.

Hormonal regulation mechanism of the sexual cycle

Mammalian reproductive processes are regulated by a complex and only partially understood cascade of combined activities from the central nervous system (CNS), several secretory tissues, target tissues and various hormones.

The CNS receives information from the animal's environment (*external, visual, olfactory, auditory, and tactile signals*) and carries this information to the hypothalamic-pituitary-ovarian axis. The hypothalamus and pituitary gland are glandular structures that are closely connected to the ventral part of the brain. They not only produce hormones but are also target organs, which creates a feedback system or homeostatic feedback. Through this feedback mechanism, most hormones regulate their own secretion rates.

Stimuli from the CNS act on the endocrine neurons of the hypothalamus to produce GnRH. This hormone is transported through the hypothalamic-pituitary portal system to the anterior lobe of the pituitary gland to secrete FSH and LH. These three hormones are released in a pulsatile manner.

FSH acts by inducing the growth and development of precavitary follicles. Then, clinically, the signs of proestrus and estrus appear. With follicular maturation, a higher level of circulating estrogens is reached and the beginning of early luteinization of the follicle is achieved, motivated by the increase in LH receptors within the follicle.

This elevation of estrogen, through positive feedback, stimulates the structures of the preoptic part to produce an ovulatory discharge of GnRH, with the consequent release of FSH and pituitary LH. LH acts by completing maturation and inducing follicle rupture by activating the ovulating enzyme complex. The control of follicular development during the cycle is done through inhibins, which are produced by the granulosa cells of the follicles themselves. They act by negative feedback on the release of pituitary FSH.

After ovulation, LH stimulates the growth of theca interna cells to form and constitute the corpus luteum (CL), hence its name luteinizing hormone.

The formed CL begins to produce progesterone, which increases its levels as the luteal tissue develops as a gland. Already in the middle of diestrus, the CL is perfectly constituted and reaches maximum progesterone production.

From the beginning of metaestrus until the end of diestrus, progesterone exerts an inhibitory or blocking action on the secretion of GnRH due to the antagonistic effect it has on sexual activity, which characterizes diestrus.

On approximately day 16 of the cycle, the CL initiates the secretion of luteal oxytocin. This hormone travels through the blood to the endometrium, where it acts by increasing and stimulating the synthesis and secretion of $PGF2\alpha$ by that organ. Then, $PGF2\alpha$ reaches the CL through the utero-ovarian circulation to cause functional lysis (luteolysis) of that gland. When CL activity ceases, serum progesterone levels drop abruptly and then the blockade it exerted on hypothalamic GnRH ceases, resuming sexual activity (*proestrus*).

Exogenous hormones

They are those that are chemically synthesized or obtained from macerates of endocrine glands of dead animals or other procedures.

Therapeutic forms to use

Therapeutic forms must consider all possibilities, but it must be considered that theoretical prognoses may be different.

The following shapes are recognized:

Substitution

The purpose of *hormone replacement therapy* is a total functional or at least phenomenological compensation of those caused by a secretory dysfunction, either due to its insufficient production or release.

Of the large number of indications, we will cite some examples: ovarian function resulting from insufficient release of LH from the pituitary (*delayed ovulation, follicular cysts*) can be successfully treated by replacement with GnRH or HCG.

What is intended is that the discharge of LH or the exogenous substitution of LH occurs so that ovulation or luteinization of the cyst occurs.

The application of progestogens for the prevention of abortion in animals that tend to abort due to dysfunction of the gestational corpus luteum is also a form of substitution.

On the other hand, estrogen replacement is of no use to intensify estrus; They can improve the intensity of heat, but do not induce ovulation.

Stimulation

With this therapy, the aim is to stimulate sexual function at rest, not very intense (*low threshold*) or also normal. As an example, let us cite the induction of heat or the provocation of superovulation with PMSG, HCG and FSH.

The hypothalamus can also be stimulated, through the positive feedback mechanism, with low doses of estrogen, so that, by rebound, it stimulates the secretion of GnRH, which in turn would produce the release of LH-FSH and thus the resumption of ovarian function.

Inhibition

The purpose of this therapy is to achieve a temporary decrease or rest in the normal functions of an endocrine gland. For example, PGF2α and its analogues inhibit the production of P_4, due to their luteolytic effect on the CL. Continued administration of progestins inhibits hypothalamic GnRH secretion and consequently blocks ovulation.

Antagonism and synergy

The lack of response from an exogenous hormone may be due to the effector organs and cells not having, at that moment of the stimulus, the specific receptors to respond to them. This may be related to the synergistic actions that are manifested between some of them. For example, estrogens induce the synthesis of oxytocin receptors in the myometrium before childbirth; if this mechanism fails, the myometrium does not respond to oxytocin, leading to primary uterine atony.

On the other hand, the chances of therapeutic success are reduced when the effector organ has undergone irreversible modifications.

An example of this is the relatively unfavorable outcome of the treatment of cystic degeneration of the ovary in dairy cows, which began to be treated three months after calving.

If the ovarian receptor cells do not respond to the direct or indirect effect of the applied hormone (LH), the limit of this therapeutic possibility has been reached.

Influence of dosage and medication idiosyncrasy

The main difficulty with hormone therapy in animals is the lack of knowledge of the exact dose required to obtain the effective response, since everyone can react differently to the same dose of a given hormone. This has to do with the animal species, breed, age, body mass and individual response threshold. Therefore, it is always recommended to use the minimum doses prescribed by the manufacturers and then check the response through a rigorous clinical examination.

Sometimes the administration of a certain hormone to an individual causes unexpected or different response from the population average, not in accordance with the dose or type of hormone. For example: a dose of 500 IU of PMSG should provoke a slight follicular development response. However, in some cows it produces moderate superovulation and in others there is no response.

All this has to do with the intrinsic characteristics of the animal when faced with drugs, the conditions of the internal environment and the true requirements of the exogenous hormone that is administered.

Preconditions for hormone therapy

The administration of hormones should only be done when it cannot be replaced by other economically profitable zootechnical actions. Other important consequences can be derived from it. For example, the apparently good effects obtained by inducing heat in poorly nourished anestric cows are short-lived and can affect the economy of the farm, since the results, in terms of number of births, are not always as expected.

Therefore, hormonal treatment of ovarian dysfunction may be contraindicated if it is not accompanied by rectifications of errors in nutrition or environmental conditions.

Hormonal treatment is indicated only when the zootechnical requirements for its successful and safe application are met. Verification that these requirements are followed requires a comprehensive clinical examination of the affected animals and the study of the causes or factors that are influencing the manifestation, to objectively evaluate the results.

It is possible that a portion of the females that have suffered from undernutrition remain in anestrus despite having increased their body mass because of improved nutrition. This is due to the lack of tonic stimulation of the endocrine system, necessary for the resumption of ovarian function. It is in these cases that hormonal stimulation treatment is indicated.

Since the administration of exogenous hormones is expensive and has its risks, the application of all these treatments must be done after a secure gynecological diagnosis. By this I mean that the use of hormones by non-professional personnel is unacceptable. Hormones are not medications to combat polyfactorial infertility in livestock, as is often claimed.

Artificial control of reproduction

GnRH analogues

In 1971 the synthesis of natural *GnRH* was achieved. Some modifications in the chemical structure of the original molecule have led to powerful analogues.

Currently there are numerous analogues created by different commercial firms including Cystorelin and Factrel (USA), Buserelin (German); Fertagyl (Dutch), Ferterelin (Japanese). Deslorelin (Australian) and Gonadorelin (Czech), Conceptal (Dutch). Ferterelin is 4-10 times more powerful than Gonadorelin and Burerelin and Deslorelin are 50 times more powerful.

It comes in the form of a lyophilized powder that must be dissolved in sterile physiological saline. Doses of 100 µg of *GnRH* analogue intramuscularly produce a response in the cow equivalent to the LH surge that precedes ovulation and increases linearly up to a dose of 1,500 µg. Intramuscular administration of 200 µg of synthetic *GnRH* causes the release of FSH and LH within 15 minutes. If the intravenous route is used, a faster response is obtained, but the amount of gonadotropin released reaches similar levels.

Indications

GnRH analogues can be used for the induction of estrus in anestric females. But the ovulatory response will depend on the presence of developing tertiary follicles, no smaller than 10 mm at the time of treatment.

They are indicated in cases of females with prolonged heat due to delayed ovulation. In higher doses they can be used effectively in the treatment of follicular and luteal cysts.

They have also been used with variable results in cows with repeat breeding syndrome attributable to failures in the maintenance of the corpus luteum by the LH.

Pituitary gonadotropins

FSH

Commercially it is produced from pituitary extract of sows, sheep, and cattle. There are different commercial preparations such as FSHp Shering (USA), Sigma (USA), Folltropin V (Canada), Superov AUSA (Australia) etc. Among them there are differences in terms of the LH content, which causes variations in the results and in terms of the dosage forms, which can be presented in mg AS (Amour Standard) or in mg NHI (National Health Institute) or equivalents in NHI units (lmg AS = 10 mg NHI).

FSHp has a wide range in the FSH-LH relationship, which constitutes a source of variation in the superovulatory response. Several studies have shown in cattle that a high LH content in FSH extracts adversely influences the effects of the ovarian response. However, a minimum amount of LH is also essential for good effects to be achieved.

Currently, a purified FSHp is being produced commercially that contains a very low proportion of LH, which makes it more effective in causing superovulation in the cow.

FSH is conserved in lyophilized form and should only be reconstituted in physiological saline solution. Due to its high protein content, it should not be dissolved in distilled water or frozen and thawed repeatedly, as there is a risk that the proteins that make it up will be hydrolyzed and the preparation will be inactivated.

For this reason, care must be taken with hygiene when handling it (needles, syringes, vials, etc.) since it can easily become contaminated.

Due to its short biological half-life, FSH must be administered every 12 hours, which guarantees the level of ovarian stimulation necessary for a certain period (4 days).

To facilitate its application, it is best to make a dilution of one mg: one ml of FSH: SSF and take the volumes corresponding to each dose (8 doses) to be administered in disposable syringes and keep them frozen so that only the dose to apply.

Oxytocin

Pituitary-derived oxytocin exerts a powerful contractile effect on uterine muscles previously sensitized by estrogen, particularly during or immediately after childbirth. It acts in the mammary gland by contracting the myofibrils of the glandular acini and the excretory ducts for the ejection of milk.

Indications

It is indicated in the treatment of primary uterine hypo or atony. An initial dose is administered IM. If after an hour of waiting there is no contractile response, the injection of the same dose should be repeated.

If after one hour of this second dose labor does not begin, the effector organ has become refractory and then there is an absolute indication for a cesarean section.

Oxytocin can be used to promote the expulsion of the retained placenta and lochia only in cases of very recent births since the uterus must be sensitized by estrogens.

The dose of oxytocin for cows and mares is 20-25 IU and for small species 5 to 10 IU via IM or subcutaneously.

Extrapituitary gonadotropins

Equine Chorionic Gonadotropin (eCG) or Pregnan Mare Serum Gonadotropin (PMSG)

This hormone originates in the trophoblast that covers the endometrial calyces of the placenta of mare. The biological activity of this chorionic gonadotropin is like that of FSH. Internationally, laboratories sell it under different names: Folligon, Intervet (France); Prianting and Shering (Germany); PMSG, Labiofam (Cuba). It is produced and packaged in lyophilized form, so its reconstruction with physiological saline solution is necessary.

It is recommended to use volumes of 5 to 10 ml so that, if there are losses during handling or injection, the calculated dose is not affected. Once the dose to be applied has been prepared, it must be used immediately. If there are leftovers, they can be kept frozen, but they should not be defrosted more than once. The way of administration is deep intramuscular, in a single dose.

Indications

Serum chorionic gonadotropin has the same therapeutic indications as pituitary FSH extracts, with the practical advantage of requiring only one treatment and having a lower cost. It is sold in one ml bulbs containing one thousand IU of the product. The dosage depends on the size of the animal and the condition being treated.

Induction of heat in the cow

The most effective treatment for the induction of heat in anestric cows in good physical condition is to inject, via IM, 50 mg of progesterone three times with 48 hours' intervals. This is done so that progesterone acts by reducing the threshold of response to serum chorionic gonadotropin.

Pass 48 hours after the last treatment, 500 to 600 IU of PMSG are injected IM. 65 to 70 % of treated cattle females should present complete heat syndrome within 24 to 36 hours following treatment.

Sometimes 10-15 % of treated cattle females have an ovarian response, but do not show psychological signs of heat. For this reason, those that are not in heat should also be inseminated, 24 and 36 hours after the last treatment.

Human chorionic gonadotropin or hCG

It is produced in the cytotrophoblast of pregnant women and due to its low molecular weight, it is excreted through urine. Its chemical structure and biological activity are like that of LH, but its biological half-life is longer than the latter.

It is sold in lyophilized form in one ml bulbs containing one thousand IU of the product so, in its preparation, the same care must be followed as with PMSG. The dosage depends on the size of the animal and the condition being treated.

Indications

It can be used, in combination with PMSG, for the induction of estrus in female bovines to ensure ovulation. It is used alone in cases of the presence of persistent follicles (prolonged heat) and for the luteinization of follicular cysts.

In general, the required dose in older animals' ranges between 1,500 to 2,000 IU. In minors it depends on their body mass.

Depending on the speed of the desired effect, intravenous, IM or subcutaneous routes are used. HCG has been used at a dose of 10,000 IU on days 10 to 12 after A.I. in the treatment of repeat breeding syndrome in cows with very variable results.

Synthetic progestogens

Under this name are grouped a whole series of synthetic compounds whose ways of acting are very different, but which have some of the properties of progesterone. These products are the basis of current contraception methods in human medicine; Their use is justified in the treatment of some forms of sterility, and they are used in veterinary medicine to induce and obtain the grouping of heat in heifers and cows.

Progestogens have the structure of cyclopentane-perhydrophenanthrene as a base; The substitutions or additions of various hydroxyl groups (OH), ketone (O), methyl (CH_3), halogens (Cl, F), in various positions have provided a whole series of products with complex actions, some of which are sometimes far from those of natural progesterone. The activity of the various progestins can be enhanced by the addition of very small amounts of estrogens.

Progesterone (P_4)

A natural progesterone dissolved in oil is sold on the market at a concentration of 10 mg/ml and packaged in 50 and 100 ml bottles. The route of administration is IM or subcutaneous and the dose will depend on the body mass of the cattle female.

Indications

Threat of abortions or repetitions of services due to CL dysfunction, hyperestronism and to enhance the activity of serum gonadotropin in the induction of heat in anestric cows, as described above.

Estrous grouping with intravaginal devices

The most effective therapeutic systems to achieve controlled heat pooling are vaginal pessaries, intravaginal devices (PRID) and subcutaneous implants.

The function of these systems is to maintain a continuous systemic level of progesterone, like that produced by the cycle CL.

The progestogens contained in intravaginal devices are slowly absorbed through the vaginal mucosa, in the necessary quantities. In this way an artificial luteal phase is created.

Removal of the device is equivalent to what happens after luteolysis, already described.

A vaginal pessary

Consists of a polyurethane sponge impregnated with a natural or synthetic progestogen in the dosage determined for each product. The sponge is inserted deep into the vagina and removed after several days by pulling a string that serves as a guide.

This pessary has the difficulty that many times they are not retained because they produce tenesmus by acting as a foreign body and in other cases, they produce purulent exudates.

The intravaginal device (PRID)

Abbott Laboratories produced a stainless steel coil (3.2 cm x 30.5 cm) covered with silicone rubber impregnated with natural progesterone. This pessary was designated **PRID** (*progesterone releasing intravaginal device*).

The large surface area of the PRID allows sufficient absorption of progesterone to maintain blood levels of P_4 that inhibit estrus. This device, with a diameter of 5 cm, is inserted into the vagina with the help of a speculum.

The presentation of estrus occurs 48 to 72 hours after being removed and the time it remains in the vagina is 10 to 14 days.

It also has the disadvantage of acting as a foreign body and producing isolated muco-purulent exudates and sometimes loss of the guides for their extraction.

To remove it, a nylon cord is pulled that remains outside the vagina. PRID retention is more than 95 %.

The subcutaneous implant

It is a small fragment (10-15 mm) of a hydrophilic polymer impregnated with a progestin. It can be placed with a 9-gauge needle or with an implant placer, subcutaneously in the back of the ear and removed when deemed appropriate according to the product used.

The Crestar® implant system consists of a Crestar® silastic implant containing 3 mg of Norgesomet (17α-acetoxy-11β-methyl-19-norpregna-4-en2.20-dion and a 2 ml Crestar® injection, which contains 3 mg of Norgestomet and 5 mg of estradiol valerate. It is used for heat grouping in heifers and cows, cyclical and non-cyclic, in A.I. or embryo transfer programs.

The implant is removed after 9-10 days so that the blockage of the pituitary gland stops, and the new follicular phase begins. In cyclical cows, heat appears after 24 to 36 hours.

In non-cyclical ones, the effect of Norgesomet is improved if the removal of the implant is combined with an IM injection of PMSG, in doses of 500 and 600 IU, for heifers and cows respectively.

Prostaglandin F2α analogues

The generic name for natural prostaglandin is dinoprost and is marketed as tromethamine salt. Its IM luteolytic dose is 25 mg (5 ml of 5 mg/ml).

Cloprostenol is a more potent analogue than dinoprost, whose luteolytic dose via IM is 500 ug (2 ml of 250 ug/ml).

Fenoprostalene is another analogue of dinoprost that has a long half-life, 18 hours or more, which favors its use in certain disorders. Its luteolytic dose is one milligram subcutaneously (2 ml of 0.5 mg/ml).

Luprostiol is another synthetic analog whose luteolytic action is obtained with a dose of 30 mg, via IM.

Indications

PG analogues are indicated to cause luteolysis in most species, except in sheep, but can also be used as ecbolic. That is, to accentuate the contractility of the smooth muscles of the tubular genital tract. Therefore, they are effective in promoting the expulsion of the retained placenta, elimination of putrefactive lochia and purulent contents of the uterine horns.

To control heat in lactating animals, it is recommended to use cloprostenol or dinoprost, both of which have a short half-life. The use of fenoprostalene, with a longer half-life (18 hours or more) is preferred in beef cattle and dairy heifers.

For oestrous synchronization in cyclical bovine females, two treatment variants can be used.

Simple dose

IM injection of a dose equivalent to 500 µg of PG with prior trans-rectal diagnosis of a CL of 8 to 16 days. Approximately 90 % of treated female cattle come into heat between 48 and 72 hours.

Double dose

All cattle females in the group are treated with PG regardless of the time of the cycle. After the first injection, approximately 45 % of the treated cattle females will present estrus (those that were in diestrus).

The second injection will be carried out again on the entire mass. After 11 days, it will match all the females in the luteal phase (those that ovulated with the first application, plus those that were in the follicular phase or that had CL less than 8 days old, which did not respond to the first injection).

More than 90 % of castle females will be in heat after 48-72 hours after the second application of PG.

Induced calving with PGF2α or its analogues

To facilitate understanding of the way exogenous hormones act in the artificial control of childbirth, I will briefly remind you of the physiological mechanism of childbirth.

During pregnancy, the placenta produces enough progesterone to maintain pregnancy.

When the fetus is at term, labor begins due to the increase in the fetus's own production of corticosteroids.

Fetal corticosteroids, especially cortisone, increase the synthesis of estrogens and PGF2α at the level of the placentomes. PGF2α acts by drastically reducing serum P_4 levels, thereby ceasing the inhibitory action that this hormone maintained on the contractility of the uterine muscles and establishing an estrogenic predominance. Then oxytocin and PGF2α can activate and trigger the expulsive phase of labor.

For the above reasons, the exogenous hormones PGF2α and dexamethasone can be used clinically to induce labor, quite effectively.

The main reasons for choosing partum induction are:

• Advance labor to reduce the interval between births;

• Prevent dystocias due to excessive fetal growth (Holstein breed);

• Terminate prolonged pregnancies due to dropsy of the ovular membranes or toxemia of pregnancy;

• Relieve abnormal breast edema during pregnancy (high producers);

• Obtain newborn blood serum (fetal serum substitute);

• Group deliveries in a certain period.

Induction method

Injection of a standard dose of PGF2α or its analogues, during the last week before the expected date of delivery, can effectively advance labor. Most cows will calve within 48 hours.

Between 28 % and 100 % of prostaglandin induced cows and heifers retain the placenta for at least 24 hours. The average retention is 59 %.

The procedure requires exact knowledge of the date of conception to prevent premature birth. This could significantly reduce the viability of the fetus and its chances of survival.

Induced calving with lidocaine and cloprostenol

In 1983, Preval and Brito, professors at the Dept. of Reproduction of the Faculty of Veterinary Medicine of Havana, reported the discovery of the properties of lidocaine to achieve the detachment of the fetal placenta in cases of placental retention in the cow.

In 1985, they devised a procedure to induce parturition, through deep intravaginal infusion of 40 ml of 2.5 % lidocaine, mixed with a small dose of cloprostenol. 80-90 % of induced births were achieved, with the particularity that they occurred during daylight hours. The best results were obtained with almost full-term pregnancies.

They also reported that the perfusion of 120 ml of a 2.5 % lidocaine solution into the uterus, in the first two hours following induced labor, allowed the avoidance of placental retention that usually occurs.

Dexamethasone induced calving

The exogenous glucocorticoid dexamethasone has been used to induce parturition in cows, sheep, and goats, but is less effective in mares and sows.

The IM injection of 20 mg dexamethasone 8 to 14 days before the expected calving of the cow produces a rapid and important drop in the concentration of progesterone in the blood plasma, to levels like that produced at the time of calving. This occurs between 22 and 56 hours after applying the treatment. Most females induced with dexamethasone retain the placenta, which is a therapeutic disadvantage.

Synthetic estrogens

Synthetic estrogens can produce actions like natural ones in the cattle female reproductive tract, but never match them. That is why they should be used with care and in the minimum doses required to achieve the desired effect.

Indications

Exogenous administration serves to increase the number of oxytocin receptors or to condition the myometrium for the most effective contractile response and, in addition, to dilate the cervix.

For this reason, they are indicated to promote the emptying of the occupied uterus in cases of retained placenta, pyometra, mucometra or hydrometra, in combination with oxytocin or PG analogues.

Diethylethylbestrol

Although this synthetic hormone is not a steroid, it has potent estrogenic activity, like oestrus syncestradiol, and is orally active in non-ruminant animals.

This estrogen is marketed by Labiofam under the name Estilbestrol in 2 ml vials containing 20 mg of the product dissolved in an oil vehicle.

The dose to be used in older animals' ranges between 15-30 mg IM. In minors, 0.5 to 15 mg depending on the species and size. If necessary, the dose can be repeated after 48 hours. The administration of this product produces signs of heat, but without ovulation.

Estradiol benzoate (BE)

Because this estrogen is a steroid, it has an effect closer to the natural hormone and the required doses are lower. It is packaged in 1 ml vials containing 1 mg of the product dissolved in an oily vehicle. The route of administration can be subcutaneous or intramuscular.

Induced oestrus

With doses of 0.5 mg via IM, heat can be achieved in the cow within 12 to 36 hours after treatment. In animals with good physical condition, 90 % heat can be reached, with 30 % ovulation. For this reason, it is recommended to inseminate treated females from the second spontaneous heat.

Early diagnosis of non-pregnancy

The intramuscular injection of 0.5 to 1 mg of BE via IM at 19-20 days after AI or mating, allows obtaining between 80-100 % return to heat of non-pregnant heifers or cows and an accuracy of the positive diagnosis from 67 % to 100 % approximately.

The variation in the precision of this diagnostic method is motivated by cases of embryonic mortality, long cycles, or deficiencies in the detection of heat.

Hormonal immune-neutralization

This biotechnology is based on the reduction of the concentration of biologically active hormone by binding, using specific antibodies generated by the animal itself (active immunization) or from another animal that has been previously hyperimmunized (in passive immunization), with the aim of increase productivity.

In the field of animal production, immunization has been done against somatostatin to accelerate the growth of lambs, against GnRH as a reversible alternative to surgical castration, and against ovarian steroids or inhibin, to increase the rate of ovulations.

When an antigen penetrates or is injected into the body, the immune response is the production of polyclonal antibodies directed against the different antigenic molecules of the injected material, making it practically impossible to separate them.

The humoral immune response is characterized by the appearance of the antibody in the blood and other body fluids and the cellular response by the appearance of processes directed against cells carrying antigens closely related to the immunogen on their membrane.

Antibodies can enhance or inhibit the activity of endogenous and exogenous hormones, so the immune system can be used to improve the reproductive efficiency of animals. When you want to temporarily delay the onset of puberty in beef heifers, immunization against GnRH can be practiced.

Vaxtrate is a vaccine against GnRH that is marketed to prevent unwanted pregnancies in beef cattle and lambs. This vaccine suppresses estrus for about 80 days and delays puberty in heifers between three and six months.

In males it is used to attenuate libido and aggressiveness or cause temporary immuno-castration.

Immunization against *PGF2α* suppresses luteolysis and therefore the resumption of estrous activity in heifers and sheep. In many cases the effect of immunization is reversible when antibody titers decrease below critical levels.

Active immunization against **inhibin** interrupts the negative feedback mechanism of inhibin on FSH secretion and consequently increases the ovulation rate. There is clinical evidence that immunization against inhibin improves embryonic quality and increases the number of embryos.

Immunization against PMSG

The greatest therapeutic difficulty that PMSG presents is that it has a biological half-life of 5 to 7 days in cattle. By acting on the ovaries for so many days, excessive superovulation can occur, and many follicles fail to ovulate due to premature luteinization. Along with this, plasma levels of estradiol notably increase in estrus and five days later, causing modifications in the motility of the oviduct and uterine horns, a premature decrease in the oocytes and the detachment of the membrane pellucida with the consequent degeneration of the oocyte and low fertility. To resolve these difficulties, anti-PMSG immuno-serum or a monoclonal antibody against PMSG has been used, which, by shortening its life in circulation, eliminates the undesirable effects.

Chapter 3

Evaluation of the reproductive performance of the herd

Content:
Reproductive indices. Control of records. Processing and calculation. Concept and interpretation of reproductive indices. The open cow and the problem cow.

Introduction

Normal and regular reproduction is the essential basis of profitable livestock breeding, therefore, improving or selecting for fertility and eliminating subfertility and sterility in livestock can mean a significant increase in milk or livestock production. meat.

From an economic point of view, permanent sterility is less important than low fertility, since completely sterile females are relatively rare compared to the high number of females that suffer from some temporary disorder of their reproductive function.

Therefore, it is necessary to know the factors capable of interfering with reproductive capacity, with the double objective of being able to maintain this fertility when it already exists and restore it if it has decreased or disappeared.

Reproductive indices

Reproductive indexes allow us to identify areas for improvement, set realistic reproductive goals, monitor progress, and identify problems at early stages. They can also be used to discover historical herd management problems.

The reproductive management of a herd must be a joint task between the farmer and the zootechnical veterinarian since the main objective is the optimization of reproductive results. Most indices for a herd are calculated as the average of individual performance. In small herds, evaluation of reproductive performance can shift from herd average to individual cow performance.

Reproductive status of the herd

The first assessment that must be made is related to the reproductive status of the herd, since this assessment measures the effectiveness of the actions developed in feeding, reproductive management, and veterinary care. The reproductive status of an ideal herd of one hundred cows shown below can serve as a comparative standard for evaluating any other herd. (Table 3-1).

Table 3-1 Reproductive status of the ideal herd

Reproductive status	Desirable value (%)
Lactating cows < 60 days	10 - 12
Inseminated or mating	25 - 30
Confirmed pregnancy	> 50
Open cows < 120 days	≤ 5
In puerperium	≤ 10

The group of inseminated or mating cows that have not yet been diagnosed with pregnancy is the one that has the greatest source of variation due to the variability in the fertility of the herds and the time at which the pregnancy diagnosis is made. This proportion could decrease by almost half when the diagnosis of pregnancy is made early (35-50 days). On the other hand, the frequency of monthly births should be 7 to 8, which is equivalent to a birth rate of 84-90 %.

Control of records

It is obvious that, to process and evaluate the reproductive data of the herd, it is necessary to ensure that the dairy has good control of the reproductive performance of each female and that all data are recorded promptly and correctly on the control card, which must be carried by the inseminator technician.

This reproductive control card contains the necessary data to know the historical background of the animal, from the moment it joins the reproduction program, until each of the births it has had. The most recent events are also recorded, such as: date of the last birth, date of inseminations after each birth, date of gestation, etc.

A dairy, farm or livestock company that does not have records of productive and reproductive data of its animals, from their birth, will not be able to aspire to improve its livestock, since the selection criteria can only be obtained from measurement and the recording of those data, in a lasting manner.

Obtaining and calculation

It must be kept in mind that no reproductive index alone allows us to reach a definitive conclusion about what is happening in the herd, so it is necessary to obtain and evaluate them as a whole and interpret their interrelationships.

Reproductive indices can be calculated, from the primary data obtained from each individual card, manually, with a digital calculator.

Although manual calculation is laborious and cumbersome, especially when the herd is larger than 50 animals, it is a feasible option to use.

It is best to do it between two people, one looks for the data on the card and the other writes down the data in a model created for this purpose.

If it is about evaluating the reproductive data of a farm or livestock company, it is most convenient to use computerized programs or applications, recognized for their simplicity and effectiveness.

If you do not have these programs, you can use the Microsoft Excel spreadsheet, in the versions of the Microsoft Office operating system available.

This application provides communication facilities to the user since it includes a general help system and does not require extensive programming knowledge. In addition, it facilitates the performance of mathematical operations through formulas and numbers stored in the "electronic cells" that can be used repeatedly to analyze the sensitivity of the input data.

Interpretation of reproductive indices

Interval calving first service (*ICFS*)

It is the time, in days, between birth and the first insemination or mating. It often coincides with the first postpartum estrus and is the one that is generally recorded on reproduction control cards. Its analysis allows us to infer how females are responding reproductively to the feeding and handling conditions to which they are subjected (postpartum anestrus) and gives an early idea of the duration of the birth-gestation period.

Uterine involution and its relationship with interval calving first estrus (*ICFE*)

The duration of uterine involution depends on many conditions: quality of diet, milk production, age, birth process, puerperium, etc.

It has been confirmed that, in general, puerperal uterine involution varies between 30 to 50 days and at the time of the first heat it is almost complete.

The incorporation of the cow into a new reproductive cycle depends on the resumption of the estrous cycle, which generally begins with the appearance of the first postpartum estrus.

It has been observed that the first postpartum estrus in dairy cows occurs between 4 to 6 weeks, on average, and in beef cows between 4 to 7 weeks and more. However, in well-fed dairy cows the first heat can appear as early as 7-15 days postpartum, a date when uterine involution has not yet been completed. This means that the cow should not be inseminated or mounted before 50 days.

This period in which uterine involution takes place is called, in livestock jargon, recentinage and the cow in this state is the recentin. So, in livestock practice, recentinage is used as a reproductive category. The rest of the reproductive categories are inseminated, gestated and empty cows.

The voluntary waiting period and the ICFS

Voluntary waiting is the period, in days, that the man decides he should wait so that the cow must be inseminated or mating after calving. This waiting period can coincide or exceed the completion of uterine involution, which normally occurs between 45-50 days. The voluntary waiting time is quite short, considering that the female reaches her highest fertility potential after 60-70 days postpartum. If the cow is inseminated 60 days postpartum.

The cows go to the inseminated category. If that inseminated cow does not return to service, or what is the same, she does not come into heat again, it is assumed that she is pregnant, but she does not move to the pregnant category until pregnancy is confirmed. This is done through rectal examination, three months after insemination or mating.

Once the pregnancy is confirmed, the cow is then placed in the category of pregnant and is given a mark as such, to differentiate it from the rest. If after 50 days the cow is not in heat (anestrus), she is then placed in the empty category.

The category of open cow depends on the duration of the period considered as postpartum physiological sexual rest, in a certain genotype and the availability of food available to supply the herd.

Nutritional and management factors influencing the duration of ICFS

The return of the estrous cycle after calving depends on internal and external factors which can act individually or in combination.

High milk production contributes to increasing ICFS length. Cows, during their maximum production, suffer an energy imbalance as they cannot have the necessary nutrients that the diet provides them and must take them from organic reserves. This causes a decrease in their body mass.

During lactation, the secretion of PIF decreases and with it that of LH-RH, with the consequent restriction of pituitary gonadotropins, thus affecting follicular maturation and ovulation.

Regarding the milking system, it has been observed that cows subjected to a 4-daily milking regime have an average interval calving-first estrus (ICFE) of 69 days, while those milked twice have heat around the 46 days.

Cows that nurse their calves can achieve ICFE averages of 72 days. This is related to the mechanism for regulating lactation and sexual functions already mentioned.

The presence of the calf with the mother also influences the maintenance of milk production. The separation of the calf or its early death modifies the lactogenic neuro-hormonal guideline complex with the consequent rapid appearance of sexual activity. This is observed in some meat breeds, and especially in the zebu, which when breastfeeding their offspring, delay the first postpartum estrus, which considerably lengthens their ICFS.

The level of postpartum feeding also closely coincides with the duration of the ICFE. Dairy cows with a high level of nutrition come into heat earlier than those with an insufficient nutritional level. The decisive factor - regarding the resumption of the estrous cyclic function after childbirth - is the preservation of the constant body condition of the mothers.

There is a close relationship between the ICFE and the ICFS, since in practice what is recorded on the cards is the ICFS, especially when the voluntary waiting period is completed. The ICFS analysis allows us to know how females are responding reproductively to the exploitation and management conditions to which they are subjected and gives us an early idea of the duration of the calving-gestation interval.

Physiological postpartum anestrus period

It is the absence of estrus, since the cow calves, until the current date. It is obtained by counting the days from the date of the last delivery to the current day. The figure obtained in this way indicates the real time that the animal has been without sexual activity and serves to assess the individual and collective situation of the herd in the face of agro-ecological, exploitation and management conditions and take the appropriate measures to shorten it.

If the prevailing environmental conditions are unfavorable or there are problems with food availability or poor management, it is expected that the return to sexuality will be delayed and postpartum anestrus will occur, prolonged. The duration of postpartum physiological rest therefore depends on the conditions.

By determining the ICFS and organizing it into a frequency distribution, one can know, retrospectively, the duration of recent past anestrus and its incidence. Apart from *Bos indicus* breeds, in well-fed cows of any genotype, anestrus of less than 60 days can be considered physiological.

In those that receive a medium level of nutrition, anestrus of up to 90 days is common. Postpartum anestrus of more than 90 days indicates the existence of a negative energy balance in the female, which prevents the resumption of ovarian activity.

Interval calving conception (ICC

It is the time between the last birth and insemination or fertilizing mating. This index is also known as service period or open days, but these names lead to confusion among non-experts.

The ICC is one of the indices that has the most predictable value, since its obtaining includes the duration of the ICFS, plus the days that the females needed to be fertilized; That is, it measures the degree of fertility that the female had after the inseminations carried out.

A short ICFS, with a long ICC, indicates that service repetitions have occurred, while a long ICFS, with an ICC equal to or slightly greater than the ICFS, indicates that anestrus has occurred. The duration of ICC should not be calculated from the number of services per conception, since the intervals between inseminations are generally longer than the duration of the normal sexual cycle (18-21 days).

Calving interval (CI)

It is the time between two consecutive births and is used to measure a cow's ability to produce a live calf in the shortest possible time.

The ideal for a rancher is that his cows can have an CI as short as 365 days, which is equivalent to obtaining one calf per year. But for this to happen, the ICC must not exceed 90 days. A longer calving interval results in longer lactation and a longer dry period.

A longer calving interval results in longer lactation and a longer dry period. Although milk production per lactation increases, milk production per year decreases since production is greater at the beginning than at the end of lactation.

Conception Services (CS)

It is also known as the insemination rate or coital rate. Expresses the number of services necessary to obtain a recognized pregnancy. The term "services" properly refers to heat, regardless of the number of inseminations or mating carried out in that heat; That is, if a cow is inseminated or mating two or three times in the same heat and because of these inseminations, she becomes pregnant, the CS number of that cow is one, since it is counted as a single service.

To calculate it, all the services received by the cattle females are added over a period of one year and divided by the number that became pregnant. Keep in mind that heifers should not be mixed with cows.

In general, heifers have a higher fertility potential than cows and consequently CS reach an average value of 1 to 1.2. If a high percentage of heifers require more than two services per conception, low quality of the semen used or problems with the application of the A.I. technique should be suspected.

In *Bos taurus* cows inseminated in Cuba, averages of 1.6 to 2.7 services/conception and 1.3 to 1.8 are reported in zebu and their crosses.

Conception rate at first service

This index also measures the fertility potential of the bull, but above all, the technical efficiency of the inseminator, who is the one who applies biotechnology. This is why it is important to know the range of normal fertility potential of the different genotypes in the country.

To calculate it, all the females that were pregnant at the first service or mating for the first time after giving birth are added, multiplied by one hundred and divided by the total number of females inseminated for the first time. A pregnancy rate at first service of more than 70 % is considered excellent, 70 % as good, 51-60 % as acceptable and less than 50 % as bad.

Inseminating technicians will be able to have good technical efficiency if they take into account important aspects such as: not giving a single service, inseminating at appropriate times, using the detector bull to know if the female is in the receptive phase of heat, not inseminating cattle females that are not are really in heat, respecting the voluntary waiting period, depositing the semen inside the cervical canal, do not use semen in poor condition, among others.

Conception rate

This indicator determines the percentage of females diagnosed as pregnant, of the total herd. It is obtained by dividing the pregnant females by the total number of the herd. The result is multiplied by one hundred. This indicator has limited utilitarian value.

Birth rate

This parameter is the one that best measures the reproductive performance of the herd, because it reveals the result of all other reproductive indices, which is the obtaining of calves born alive.

There are two ways to calculate it depending on whether heifers are included.

$$\text{Birth rate} = \frac{\text{N. of calves born alive} \times 100}{\text{Average number of cows on farm}}$$

$$\text{Birth rate} = \frac{\text{N. of calves born alive} \times 100}{\text{N. of cows} + 50\% \text{ of heifers over 18 months old}}$$

For the exploitation conditions of tropical livestock, it is preferable to use the first form, since the age at which the heifers start breeding varies greatly in the different genotypes and livestock farms.

For dairy cattle, a birth rate of 80 % is excellent, 70 % or more is good, more than 60 % is acceptable, and less than 50 % is bad.

For zebu cattle, under conditions of extensive breeding and free riding, a birth rate of 70 % is excellent, 64 % is good, and less than 50 % is bad.

Rate of non-births

It is given by the percentage of females considered pregnant that should have given birth and do not do so due to abortions, diagnostic errors, and deaths. It should not be more than 3-5 %.

When this percentage exceeds 5 %, possible conflicts of interest should be suspected in technical personnel who receive a better salary when they report more females as pregnant. The professional must be alert to the commission of fraud in the records, especially when many abortions and diagnostic errors are reported.

The open cow and the problem cow

This term means that the female is in a more or less transitory unproductive phase. It includes both the time of functional postpartum anestrus and eventual infertility due to repetitions of service. Consequently, the open cow is undesirable from an economic and statistical point of view, especially when it remains in that state for a long time. The empty cow may or may not be infertile.

The open infertile cow is called a "*problem cow*"; For example, cows that do not conceive after having received three services from A.I. are designated as "*problems*", they are separated from the herd and mated with the so-called fourth heat bulls. These are measures that have no scientific basis. First of all, when artificial insemination is applied, natural mating is contraindicated. Secondly, if the supposedly infertile cow becomes pregnant by the bull, it means that that cow was not actually infertile.

Chapter 4

Comparative genital anatomy and physiology

Content:
Gonadal and uterine anatomical differences. Ovaries of the *Bos taurus*. Ovaries of *Bos taurus indicus* and their crosses. Anatomical and functional characteristics of the corpus luteum. Uterus. Fundamental and common physiological processes in all races. Heat detection. Proestrus. Oestrus. Clinical diagnosis of pregnancy. Ultrasound diagnosis.

Introduction

Knowledge of the anatomical and functional characteristics of the reproductive system of female cattle is essential for the clinician to be able to correctly interpret the reproductive processes and not make diagnostic errors. This is particularly true when the genital anatomy and physiology of European *Bos taurus* females is compared with *Bos taurus indicus* (zebu) and it is found that there are notable differences in some of their organs and systems.

Absorbent crosses between *Bos taurus* bulls and zebu females lead to the improvement of dairy or meat qualities, but some undesirable traits of zebu cattle, particularly in the reproductive area, are transmitted to the offspring, to one extent or another, and must be considered.

Gonadal and uterine anatomical differences

Ovaries of the *Bos taurus*

In heifers of this species, the ovaries exceed the size of a large bean or peanut; In cows, the gonads average 3-4 cm in length, about 2.5 cm in width and 1.5-2.0 cm in thickness; Its size varies from a pigeon's egg to a dwarf chicken's egg. Its shape is ovoid, acute towards the uterine extremity.

Size and shape of the ovaries of *Bos indicus* cattle

In the literature consulted, variations are reported in the average values of the diameter of the right and left ovaries between the different breeds of *Bos indicus* cows: 3.0 and 1.69 cm for Brazilian zebu; 2.56 and 2.50 cm for the Thari; 2.62 and 2.5 cm for the Nelore and 2.3 and 1.10 cm: for the Gir.

In cyclic Fulani cows, the left ovary was found to be shorter, narrower and less heavy than the right. Small, rounded ovaries were considered abnormal, that is, atrophied or hypoplastic.

However, through numerous observations carried out over several years, we were able to verify that these reported biometric values did not coincide with the measurements that we obtained from the ovaries of the Bos indicus females studied.

New findings on the ovarian biometry of *Bos indicus* and its crosses with *Bos taurus*

In crossbred heifers and zebu cows, we discovered the existence of three types of ovaries, which differ in size and shape. Small and rounded, about the diameter of a pea (0.8 to 1 cm); medium and ovoid, (2-3.5 cm), and large flattened, (5-6 cm), (Fig. 4-1 and 4-2). Heifers and cows of the Cuban zebu breed have a greater frequency of the type of ovaries small, but not the type with large, flattened ovaries, characteristic of zebu crossbreeds.

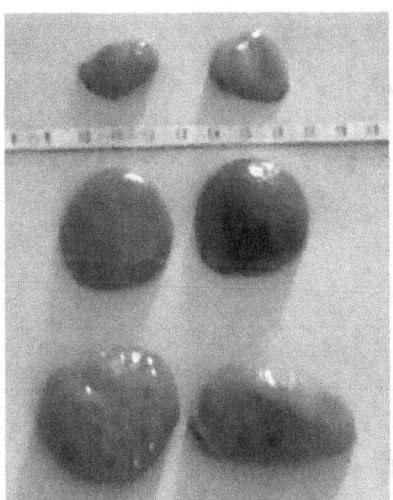

Fig. 4-1 Ovaries of zebu cows   Fig. 4-2 Heifer ovaries

Figure 4-1 shows six inactive ovaries of zebu cows. Note the size difference among them.

Figure 4-2 shows a zebu heifer genital tract with large, flattened inactive ovaries. Two small ovaries were superimposed for comparison.

From the second F_2 generation of the Holstein x Zebu crossbreeding, the type of large, flattened ovary decreases until it almost disappears; but the small ovary type remains at a high frequency (Table 4-1).

It is of clinical interest to know that these three types of ovaries can also be found in heifers, although the large, flattened ovary in heifers is somewhat smaller than in cows (Figure 4-2). Note that in that figure I placed two small ovaries on top of the large ones to serve as a comparison. I clarify that these measurements were made directly with a caliper to inactive ovaries, without the presence of tertiary follicles or corpora lutea that would alter their size in any way.

Twenty-nine percent of Siboney cows may have ovaries as small as 10 mm in diameter, very difficult for non-experts to palpate. In general, in this new breed there is a predominance of small ovaries (15-20 mm).

Table 4-1 Ovary size of Holstein x zebu cows

Crossbreeding	10 mm		15-20 mm		25-30 mm	
	n	%	n	%	n	%
½ H x ½ C (F_1)	0,0	0,0	26	32,0	43	54,0
¾ H x ¼ C (F_2)	33	33,0	55	55,0	12	12,0
⅝ H x ⅜ C (F_3)	30	29,0	77	58,0	18	13,0
⅞ H x ⅛ C (F_4)	28	24,0	66	56,0	24	20,0
Legend: Very smalls (10 mm); smalls (15-20 mm); medium (25-30 mm)						

Ovarian biometry of Ethiopian Boran cows (*Bos indicus*)

The Boran breed is considered the mother breed of the African zebu. It is native to the Boran Plateau in southern Ethiopia. Due to its rusticity, tameness and productive qualities, it is the most widespread breed on the African continent.

In this breed we were also able to verify the existence of very small, small and medium ovaries

Table 4-2 shows the results of ovarian biometry performed on a group of 64 Ethiopian Boran cows. 54 % of the left ovaries had a size of 1,0 to 1,5 cm in diameter. 44 % of the right ovaries were 1,0 to 1,5 cm in diameter. The maximum value reached was 4 cm in diameter.

Table 4-2 Size of ovaries of Boran cows, according to its largest diameter

Size en cm	Left ovary		Right ovary	
	n	%	n	%
1,0 – 1,5	35	54,0	26	44,0
2,0 – 2,5	27	42,0	32	50,0
3,0	2	4,0	4	6,0

Holstein x Boran crossbred cows

The overall average size of the ovaries of crossbred Boran cows was 2,3±0,4 cm and 2,7±0,6 cm, for the left and right respectively. The amplitude of variation in the left ovary was 1 to 3 cm and 1,0 to 3,5 cm in the right. 52.4 % of the cows left ovaries had a size of 1,0 to 1,5 cm in diameter. 20.0 % of the cows' right ovaries had a diameter of 1,0 to 1,5 cm.

The results of the gonadal biometry performed on Ethiopian Boran cows and their crossbreeding with *Bos taurus* highlight peculiarities of ovarian size that differentiate them from the rest of the zebu breeds observed, not only because of the small size of their ovaries, but also because of their high incidence.

Another peculiarity is that ovaries of the large, flattened type like those observed in the cross-bred zebu cows from Cuba were not found.

No statistical association was found between the size and shape of the ovaries and their reproductive fitness, weight, or age. The fact that the types of ovaries described can be found in both prepubertal heifers and in adult, old, recently calved, and pregnant cows confirms that the small ovary type is a characteristic anatomical trait of the subspecies *Bos taurus indicus*, which is transmitted to through inheritance.

Anatomical and functional characteristics of the corpus luteum

Evolution of the corpus luteum (CL)

The corpus luteum is formed from the granulosa cells of the theca interna of the ovulated follicle. During the 3-4 days after ovulation, the follicular cavity is filled with large and small thecal cells that become luteal cells, which give rise to the corpus luteum. During the days that follow, the CL begins to become protuberant and slightly exceeds the ovarian surface. Clinically it is possible to palpate the CL after the 5th to 6th day of the cycle. At the beginning of its development, the CL that protrudes from the surface of the ovary is small, but it quickly increases in size and reaches its maximum development after 7-16 days of the cycle. Fig. 4-3 shows seven ovaries with corpora lutea at different stages of development.

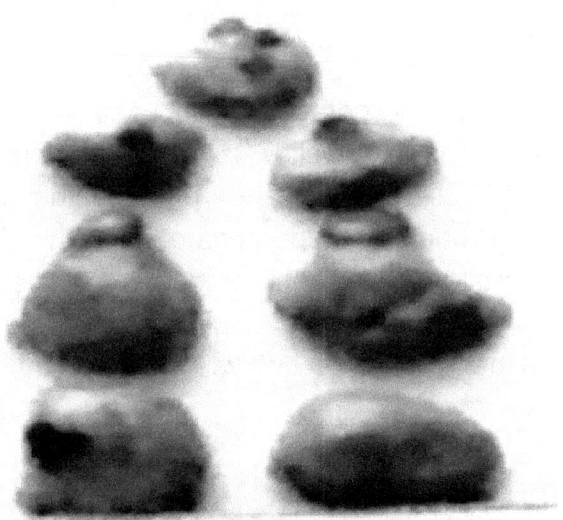

Fig. 4-3 Ovaries with CL in different stages

The prominent part of the CL forms a solid button of soft consistency that can vary in height (0,5 to 1 cm), but sometimes the CL does not appear prominent and is completely included within the ovary. Since the CL reaches a diameter of 2,5-3 cm^2, it can modify the size and shape of the ovary in question. For example, when the CL develops in one pole of the ovary, it takes an elongated shape; When it develops in the middle part, it can take on a triangular shape, like a Y or an L.

These modifications in shape and size, together with the change in consistency, are important elements to be able to differentiate, clinically, the presence of a rounded mass of a semi-hard consistency included in the ovary.

When it comes to zebu females, which can have ovaries of 1 to 2 cm in diameter, the CL covers a larger surface than the ovarian parenchyma itself.

It is curious that the corpus luteum continues to retain its original name due to its yellow color, like the pigment lutein found in plants, algae, and photosynthetic bacteria. However, this name is inappropriate since the CL is a true internal secretion gland that produces progesterone and oxytocin and not a simple body included in the ovary. Regarding the color, it is not yellow either but rather red orange.

Involution of CL

When the ovulated oocyte is not fertilized for any reason, the periodic or cycle CL begins to undergo regression or involution, starting on day 16 of the cycle. This regression is associated with the pulsatile release of PGF2α, produced in the endometrium.

The mechanism of how PGF2α acts on the luteal gland, suppressing its functioning, is not well clarified, but in the scientific literature it is known as luteolysis. For non-specialists, the word luteolysis can be interpreted as dissolution or decomposition of the corpus luteum, but that is not what really happens. What happens is: on day 16 of the cycle, uterine PGF2α reaches the CL and produces general vasoconstriction that suppresses its secretory activity.

The serum progesterone concentration decreases drastically, the follicular phase resumes and the female goes into heat. However, the structure of the CL persists morphologically in the ovary, without undergoing major changes.

This means that, at the time of the new cycle, the preceding CL is present without influencing the sexual function of the following cycles. Thus, the involution of the CL is a slow and gradual process, in which the luteal gland changes size, consistency and color, until it becomes an impalpable scar.

In general, after 28-30 days from the beginning of the infertile cycle, the remains of the CL can be palpated on the surface of the ovary as a hard formation the size of a chickpea. These formations allow the clinician to recognize that the animal is cycling or has recently done so.

Histologically, the involution of the CL is characterized by the replacement of thecal cells by fibrous connective tissue. As involution progresses, the size reduces and there is a change in color towards red (*corpus rubrum*), until it becomes a whitish scar formation, called *corpus albicans*, after several months.

Uterus

No differences are reported in the anatomy and physiology of the uterus of both subspecies, although the size of the uterine horns of Bos taurus females tends to be more voluminous and heavier with age. On the other hand, notable differences are seen in the cervix.

Cervix of Bos taurus

In these females the cervix has a cylindrical and elongated shape, in heifers it is 8 to 10 cm long and 1,5 to 2,0 cm in diameter; In cows it increases both in thickness (3-4 cm) and length (10-15 cm) depending on age and number of births.

Cervix of Bos indicus

In a relatively high percentage of zebu cows, a manifest thickening of the cervix can be observed, caused by hyperplasia of the collagen tissue that makes up the structure of the cervix. In these cases, the cervix takes the shape of a funnel and dilates at the back. The neck can become the thickness of a fist and even the size of a child's head, difficult to grasp with the hand inserted into the rectum; they are often curved in a U or S shape.

In *crossbred zebu heifers* the length of the cervix ranges from 3,4 to 8,5 cm, with an average of 5,8 cm. The number of transverse rings varies from 3 to 5. The shape of the cervix is straight and normally, the cervical canal is patent.

In *cows*, the length of the cervix ranges from 4,7 to 13,5 cm, with an average of 8,4 cm. The shape of the cervix is straight in 55 % of cows; but 45 % show curved cervices. Normally the cervical canal is patent.

In general, Zebu heifers have small, straight cervices. On the other hand, in cows they are of different sizes; small, (2 cm in diameter); medium (3-4 cm) and large (more than 4 cm in diameter), and due to their shape, they can be straight, slightly curved and curved in a U or S (See Fig.4-4).

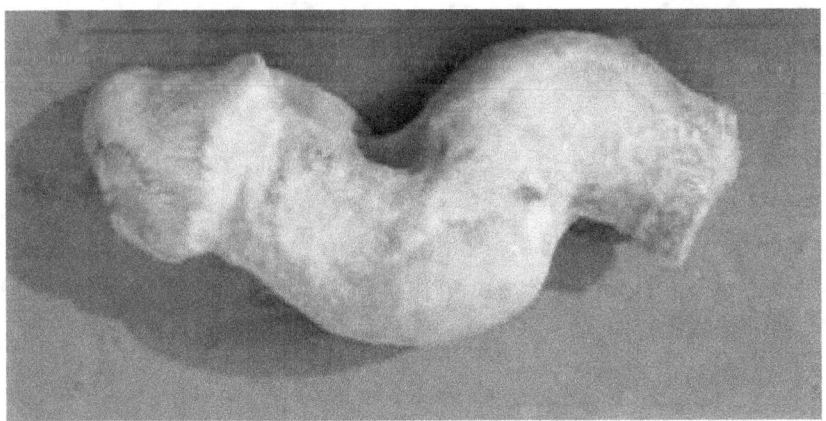

Fig. 4-4 S-shaped curve of the cervix

As in the ovaries, there is a predominance of the medium cervix and a smaller percentage of the large one. The proportion of straight cervix is only 50 %.

Santa Gertrudis breed cows, which have *Bos taurus indicus* genes in their genotype, also have enlarged cervices. Sometimes the organ can be so large that it can barely be covered and grasped with the hand inserted into the rectum.

Boran cows from Ethiopia have:

a) Small cervices (56 %)

b) Medium cervices (34 %)

c) Large cervices (10 %)

Regarding their shape, 73,4 % are straight and 27,0 % are curved.

In absorbent crosses of crossbred Holstein x zebu cows, the three cervice sizes reported in Bos taurus indicus cows are also found, but the presence of medium and large and curved necks tends to decrease with the absorption of Bos taurus genes (Table 4-2).

Table 4-2 Frequency distribution of the cervical biometry in cows Holstein x Zebu crossbreeds

Size and shape	Absorbent crossover degree							
	F1		F2		F3		F4	
	n	%	n	%	n	%	n	%
Small and straight	27	34,4	64	64,0	67	59,0	80	67,0
Medium and straight	20	24,6	20	20,0	29	26,5	4	3,4
Medium and stooped	20	24,6	6	6,0	7	7,5	14	11,8
Big and straight	8	10,0	4	4,0	6	4,5	14	11,8
Big and hunched	5	6,4	----	-----	4	2,5	6	5,0

Despite this, neither cervical enlargement nor U and S shaped deformations produce strictures or obstructions of the cervical canal and, consequently, do not prevent fertilization, pregnancy, or childbirth. However, when the deformations are very pronounced, they make it impossible for any catheter to pass into the body of the uterus. This difficulty must be considered when selecting zebu and Santa Gertrudis cows as embryo donors or recipients.

Physiological processes in all breeds

Clinical detection of estrus

Where artificial insemination or hand mating is being used, oestrus detection is the most important limiting factor for optimum reproductive performance. However, this task is frequently not given due attention.

Deficiencies in the detection of estrus can be one of the causes of the prolongation of the service period and therefore the increase in economic losses due to non-productive days.

Given that in the sexual cycle of the bovine female the proestrus, estrus and metaestrus periods have some clinical peculiarities that can make their identification difficult, it is advisable that the professional and technical personnel recognize their clinical symptoms well, so that this knowledge can be transmitted to the people in charge of monitoring estrus.

The proestrus

In proestrus, the follicular activity of the ovaries resumes and estrogens stimulate the hypothalamic sexual center, producing some modifications in the genital tract and in the psychic behavior of the animal.

As proestrus progresses, some secondary symptoms may appear, such as slight swelling of the vulva, excretion of crystalline or opaque vaginal mucus, abundant, not very viscous, and frequent mooing.

However, the appearance of the reflex of jumping and hugging towards other cattle females is the most striking sign for the clinical recognition of advanced proestrus. Whenever the observer sees a cattle female jumping on another, he should identify her by her ear number and continue observing her for several minutes to see if she continues to repeatedly jump on the same or another cow. If the cattle female jumps on others indiscriminately, it is she who is in proestrus; If a cow jumps on another more than once, the one that is in heat is not the one that jumps but the one that is being ridden, since it expresses the reflex of tolerance to jumping and hugging.

Estrus or heat

When a female bovine is mounted by a bull or another cow and remains immobile firmly on all fours, she is manifesting the *standing reflex*. This reflex is the main indicator of heat or estrus and means that the female is suitable to be mating by the bull or instrumentally inseminated. Another sign that characterizes this period is the cervico-vaginal mucous secretions that become more abundant and extensible, capable of forming long threads and that smear the vulva and perineal region of the animal.

Along with the various symptoms that appear during proestrus and estrus, the production of *pheromones* is activated by the action of circulating estrogens. The function of this chemical substance is to attract the male and for him to recognize her for mating. When the bull perceives the smell of the pheromone present in the cervico-vaginal mucus and that marks the urine and feces of the female in heat, the Flehmen reflex is activated.

Flehmen reflex consists of a particular expression, in which the bull retracts its nose backwards and extends its head for a short time. But these pheromones are also perceived by the other cows in the herd, which participate by executing the jump on those that are in heat. In practice, the cows in the herd are the ones that first detect heat.

To make the appropriate differentiation between a female in proestrus, another in estrus and others that act only as jumpers, the observant is required to watch over the females for at least 30 minutes, to verify the repetitiveness of the jumps.

In case of doubt, both the female that jumps and the one that allows itself to be jumped must be separated in a pen, so that the inseminator technician can carry out the internal diagnosis of heat.

The value of uterine contractility in the estrus detection

One of the causes of repeat breeding may be to inseminate the female without being in heat and this happens to inseminate technicians who do not know how to correctly identify the internal symptoms of heat.

During this period, ovarian estrogens increase the spontaneous motor activity of the smooth muscles of the uterus. Consequently, the uterine horns contract when palpated and roll in on themselves. This contraction of the horns that makes them firm and hard is called "estrus erection." So, if the uterine horns of the female in question are flaccid or relaxed, she cannot be in heat.

Another sign that can help is the presence of very extensible vaginal mucous secretions that flow through the vulva during manipulation of the vagina through the rectum, when the female is in heat.

Duration

Wide variations in the duration of estrus are reported, ranging from 6 to 30 hours. These large differences are motivated by the different ways of interpreting heat syndrome and the methods used to measure its duration.

In this book it is assumed that estrus begins when the female allows herself to be jumped and hugged and ends when she rejects the hug.

In *Bos taurus* cattle raised in a subtropical climate, an average heat duration of 12-15 hours is reported, with no differences between breeds. In zebu heifers, heat can last from 7 to 16 hours and in cows from 13 to 18 hours on average.

Other factors not associated with social behavior may influence the duration of estrus. Younger females have a shorter estrus than older females. Cold weather or prolonged rain can minimize sexual expressiveness. Environmental heat stress decreases sexual activity with a tendency to shorten heat.

Early metaestrus or postestrus

The inclusion of metaestrus in this section is because it is the transition period from the follicular to the luteal phase, with the characteristic that, in the bovine female, ovulation occurs approximately 12 hours after the end of heat, that is, in the early metaestrus.

The main sign that indicates that the cow is entering metaestrus is that it does not allow itself to be mounted. This occurs because the sexual center becomes refractory to the action of estrogen and the female stops expressing of the standing reflex.

Despite this, the Graafian follicle, with its production of estrogen, continues to be present for a few more hours, acting on the uterine receptors and activating the production of pheromones. For that reason, a bull can recognize a cow in early metaestrus, as if she were in heat.

At this stage the bull executes the jump, but the cow avoids the hug. On rectal examination, the uterine horns remain contractile, but lose the typical hardness of the estrous erection. In addition, mucous secretions become denser, grayish, and less abundant. These signs can be recognized by a competent inseminator technician.

At 35 to 45 hours after postestrus, a bloody mucus that characterizes metaestrus appears in 90 % of heifers and 50 % of cows, which is indicative that the animal was in heat. This blood comes from the rupture of some capillaries of the endometrium, caused by the sudden decrease in estrogen and has no pathological significance.

From a practical point of view, the presence of blood in the metaestral mucus can be used to know whether the artificial insemination carried out was done at a favorable time or not.

If bloody mucus appears within 24 hours after A.I. the female was inseminated very late; If it appears after 36 hours, the cow was inseminated too early. This condition can clarify, in many cases, subfertility caused by failures in the organization of directed reproduction.

Diurnal variations in the appearance of heat

In zebu females, the highest frequency of heat occurs during the day, from 9:00 AM to 3:00 PM.

In *Bos taurus*, most heat occurs between 6:00 AM and 6:00 PM. 30 to 40 % of estrus begins at night, between 9:00 PM and 12 Midnights.

This is particularly important for the rancher since, if the female has a short heat at dusk, she will end the receptive phase at dawn the next day and will not be detected in heat. This is one of the causes of apparent anestrus.

According to the above, to detect 90 % of the herd's heat, careful observation is required in the early morning and late afternoon hours.

Expressiveness of heat syndrome

The absence of a male as a biological stimulus can cause an incomplete or inadequate expression of the clinical and psychological symptoms of heat. Therefore, the inclusion of a vasectomized bull or one with a deviated penis in the herd as a social companion can influence a satisfactory expression of estrus. Additionally, females limit their expressions of heat when they are about to be milked, when they are eating, or when they are moved for cleaning. Slippery floors waterlogged and muddy pens, and other situations that make it difficult for animals to move safely affect the expressiveness of the jumping and hugging reflex.

Therefore, the best times for mating are when the cows are gathered to be transferred to the milking parlor, when they are free in the pasture grazing or ruminating, or when they are moved to the shade room.

Hours and duration of estrus detection

As the length of 20 % of heats can be less than 6 hours and as heat begins at any time of the day, it is most convenient to make three observations a day: one at 6-7:00 AM, another at 1-2:00 PM and another at 5-6:00 PM. The duration of the observations should not be less than 30 minutes since cows tolerate being mounted once every 20 minutes on average.

Detection of estrus requires without exclusion:

A) A person trained and capable of distinguishing the different symptoms of heat and the symptoms of proestrus and early metaestrus.

B) That person has enough time to observe the herd, at least twice a day.

C) That it has adequate auxiliary means for detecting heat.

a) Because the main external signs of heat in cattle are distinguishable, many believe that any cowboy can be a heat watcher. Perhaps for this reason, in the country's livestock companies the practice of training dairy staff in the technique of heat detection is neglected, which, as has been seen, is not as simple as it seems. It is recommended that the technical and professional personnel who serve the units undertake this training, as they are the most qualified to do so.

b) When dairy herds are very large, cowboys lose contact with the cows and identification of females in heat becomes very difficult. In these cases, it is indicated that a man be appointed, especially dedicated to the observation and separation of females in heat, and that he receives appropriate training.

If the herds have 25 to 50 cows, it is not justified to pay a man to monitor their heat, but then it becomes necessary for the dairy staff to assume surveillance of the open cows, at least twice a day, for 30 minutes, as already explained.

c) Different auxiliary means have been used to detect heat, but the most effective have been the bulls themselves, surgically prepared.

In this chapter we will mention the two that have shown the best results in practice.

1) Vasectomy

Which is based on surgical section of each of the vas deferens, which go along the spermatic cords at the exit of the bull's testicles. It produces sterility, with the advantage that the animal fully preserves the primary sexual reflexes.

The surgical intervention is simple, quick and requires few materials and medications to perform it. The postoperative period lasts only 3-4 weeks.

2) Surgical deviation or transplantation of the penis from the natural position

This is the technique that has been used in Cuba for many years and has allowed, together with artificial insemination, to keep the country almost free of venereal diseases.

It consists of the surgical deviation of the penis and foreskin at an angle of 45 to 50 degrees from their original position. The animal executes the jump but cannot penetrate the penis into the vagina.

To minimize the risks of postoperative complications and deaths, these deviations are performed on yearlings weighing 200 to 300 kg, which have a short foreskin.

These yearlings with deviated penises are kept separate from the females until they reach sexual maturity and are accepted by the herd as bulls and act as assistants to the heat detector man.

The transplant of the foreskin and penis is a laborious and relatively expensive operation since it requires the use of sedatives, local anesthesia, surgical material, antibiotics, and postoperative care; perhaps for these reasons it has not spread internationally.

With the materials needed to perform a penile diversion, about 15 vasectomies can be performed. However, penile diversion is the safest procedure to eradicate venereal diseases since there is no penile penetration.

Selection and management of teaser bulls

The main mission of a teaser bull is to recognize females in heat, therefore, before being incorporated into the herd, its sexual performance must be checked with the female and a series of important requirements must be met. Example: he must have reached a minimum body mass of 400 kg and a size approximately equal to that of the females he is going to detect. Otherwise, it will become a subordinate element within the social group of the herd. Hence, recently operated yearlings or steers should not be incorporated into herds until they reach the indicated body mass.

Placed in front of a female in heat, the teaser bull must be active, with repeated actions of approaching, jumping and hugging. If signs of semi-frigidity or frigidity are found (poor virility, sexual apathy), the bull must be rejected as a teaser or eliminated if it had already been incorporated as such.

With respect to this important aspect, I clarify that *Bos indicus* males should not be selected as teaser because they have a very pendulous and long foreskin and a very slow reaction time. On the other hand, *Bos taurus* males of dairy breeds and their crossbreeds with *Bos indicus* are more ardent.

After the last mating of the afternoon, it is advisable to separate the bulls from the females, so that they do not exhaust themselves by jumping uselessly during the night. Each cow detected in heat must be marked and taken to the stall.

Use of teaser bull to identify the receptive phase of estrus

In routine work, the inseminator technician does not have any objective clinical procedure that allows him to determine the most appropriate moment to perform the A.I. For this reason, the teaser bull must be assisted to check if the female is in the receptive phase of estrus. If a female is detected in heat early in the morning and shows the standing reflex, she should be inseminated that same morning. If in the afternoon she still allows herself to be mounting, she should have a second service. If heat is detected in the morning hours, it is most likely that the receptive phase will occur in the afternoon.

Verification of this fact must be done with the heat detector bull. This simple fact of using teaser bulls to check the standing reflex can help increase the fertility rate of females, reduce the number of services to obtain fertilization and make bovine exploitation more economical.

Reasons to use double service

When there is a good job of heat detection and the bull is used to check the tolerance reflex, the inseminator technician only needs to use a single service to achieve an acceptable fertility rate.

If difficulties are encountered with the detection of heat and it is suspected that a few hours have passed since its beginning (night heat), it is logical that the best results are obtained when a first service is applied as soon as the animal is detected in heat and a second 4 to 6 hours later. This is particularly true of estrus observed in the morning.

If the female is detected in heat in the afternoon, she should receive the first service in the late afternoon and early morning of the next day. A cow in prolonged heat may require a third service.

Clinical diagnosis of pregnancy

Checking the pregnancy status is essential for good reproductive management of the herd. Although several methods can be used, we will discuss here only those most used in livestock farming.

The non-return rate

It is because the sexual cycle of cattle is continuous. If several cows are inseminated and do not return to estrus after 18-21 days, it is assumed that they are pregnant. But this assumption is not accurate since some of them may not be. On the other hand, up to 7 % of cows may be in heat during the first third of pregnancy. For these reasons, the non-return to heat test is not a reliable diagnostic method.

Rectal palpation

It is the most economical, fastest, and safest method to diagnose pregnancy, even in very early stages. Rectal palpation of the uterus and its contents is a good clinical method to calculate the age of gestation.

The elements used to recognize the state of pregnancy through rectal examination are:

1- Presence of a well-developed corpus luteum in one of the ovaries

2- Location, retractility and weight of the uterus

3- Asymmetry, consistency, and fluctuation of the uterine horns

4- Presence of fetal membranes

   a) Palpation of the amniotic vesicle

   b) Palpation of the allantochorion vessels (double wall)

5- Palpation of parts of the fetus

6- Presence of placentomes

7- Hypertrophy and thrill of the middle uterine artery

Early diagnostic

The best time to safely diagnose pregnancy is at the end of the 5th week in the heifer and the 6th week in the cow. The asymmetry is recognized because one of the horns is more developed, filled with fluid, with its wall more thinned and contains the amniotic sac, which can be palpated as a turgid vesicle of 1 to 1.5 cm in diameter, floating in the allantoic fluid.

At the end of the 6th week, the asymmetry is more developed, the horn is filled with fluid and dilated. Fetal fluids and membranes penetrate further into the caudal part of the horn and into the body, thus facilitating palpation of the double wall. The pregnant horn has an average diameter of 4-6 cm and the amniotic sac 2-3 cm.

Middle diagnosis

At the end of the 7th week, the gestational horn is 5-7 cm, and the asymmetry is very marked. The uterus fills the pelvis and moves slightly into the abdominal cavity. Fluctuation, asymmetry, and double wall are clearly detected throughout the pregnant horn. The uterine body dilates in the shape of a bell. The amniotic sac is the size of a guinea egg and is gradually losing its turgidity.

At the end of the 8th week, the asymmetric uterus can retract into the pelvic cavity, there is fluctuation, the vessels of the allantochorion are palpated as a double wall, but the amniotic sac cannot be differentiated. Instead, the fetus can be palpated between the fingers, which by this time reaches 5-8 cm in length. The middle uterine artery has increased in size slightly, but there is no thrill.

Remember that thrill is the pulsating vibration that is perceived when the middle uterine artery or one of its branches is held between the fingers.

In three-month pregnancy, the changes in the uterus are easily distinguishable. The uterus moves into the abdominal cavity. At 70 days the uterus is no longer retractable. Between the 9th and 10th weeks, the pregnant uterus is the thickness of a forearm (8-12 cm). Palpating the thin uterine wall reveals placentomas the size of a black bean. If the vibration of the uterus is done, the contact of the fetus is felt by rebound.

Between the 11th and 12th weeks, the gestational horn sinks towards the abdominal cavity and reaches a volume larger than a human arm. The placentomes are palpable and measure 1.5 x 0.5 cm and when performing the ballooning the fetus is perceived against the hand. At the end of the 3rd month, the uterine artery reaches 0.5-0.7 cm in diameter, undulates in the broad ligament and transmits the arterial thrill intermittently. All the signs of pregnancy already described appear.

Late diagnosis

In the fourth month of gestation, the entire uterus descends into the abdominal cavity, drags the cervix, and prolongs the vaginal cavity, so that, in large cows, it is possible to palpate only the neck and body of the dilated uterus. The wall of the uterus is very thin and the placentomes reach the size of a large bean to a walnut (1.5 x 2.5 cm). The middle uterine artery reaches the thickness of a pencil and has a thrill.

The fifth month of pregnancy is very similar to the previous one, but the uterus is very difficult to palpate. Pregnancy is proven by the prolongation of the vagina, the impossibility of palpating the uterus and by the change in caliber of the middle uterine artery, which reaches the thickness of the little finger (0.7-0.9 cm), with the typical gestational thrill. A similar situation occurs in the sixth month of pregnancy, and it is difficult to differentiate it from the fifth.

Pregnancies from the end of the fourth month to the sixth are the most difficult to diagnose and the most prone to confusion since the uterus and its contents sink deeply into the abdominal cavity, far from the hand of the operator, who cannot palpate nothing, except the hypertrophy of the middle uterine artery, with its strong arterial vibration. For a connoisseur, these signs are clear evidence of an advanced pregnancy.

During the seventh month, the uterus begins to return toward the pelvic cavity. By inserting the hand into the rectum, the fetus is easily palpated. In the last two months of gestation, the fetus is palpated in the pelvic cavity.

The most unequivocal signs to verify pregnancy are:

a) Presence of the amniotic sac

b) Presence of the double wall or allantoic vessels

c) Presence of the fetus

d) Presence of placentomes

The clinical finding of each of these signs is sufficient to prove pregnancy. In case of doubt, it is preferable to repeat the diagnosis one to two weeks later. For not very qualified personnel, the best time to make a pregnancy diagnosis is 12 weeks since almost all the possible signs to identify a pregnancy are present currently.

Recognition, by rectal palpation, of the signs described above and that accompany the different stages of pregnancy, can be relatively easy for those who have experience in palpation of non-pregnant uteri. Therefore, the first requirement to learn to diagnose pregnancy rectally is to know how to locate and identify the internal genital organs of non-pregnant cows and heifers.

Ultrasonographic diagnosis

Ultrasonography equipment is made up of a console (monitor, keyboards, commands and mechanisms that transform electrical signals into images) and a transducer or probe (made up of piezoelectric crystals capable of vibrating due to the electrical impulses it receives and transmitting sound waves) that It is placed in direct contact with the animal, with which the operator is able to visualize organs previously accessible only through palpation on the console.

Basic concepts and generalities of ultrasonography

Ultrasonography uses high-frequency sound waves (20 Megahertz (Mhz), 1 Mhz is equivalent to 1,000,000 sound waves per minute, above the sound capable of being heard by humans).

When the Ultrasound wave interacts with tissues, different physical processes occur: Transmission, Reflection, Refraction, Dispersion, Absorption and Attenuation.

The reflected ultrasound (US) pulses detected by the transducer need amplification by the equipment (console), all this information is stored by a computer and displayed on the television (monitor).

Terms most used in ultrasound descriptions:

• **Acoustic window:** This is a tissue or structure that offers little obstacle to the penetration of sound waves, and therefore can serve to obtain images of deep structures. For example, a bladder full of urine allows a better view of pelvic structures.

• **Anechogenic:** These are structures without echoes, or echo-free (e.g. liquids).

• **Hyperechogenic or hyperechoic:** These are tissues that cause brighter echoes than neighboring tissues, for example bones, perirenal fat, etc.

• **Hypoechogenic *(hypoechoic)*:** These are tissues that cause a reduction in the intensity of the echoes, when compared to neighboring tissues, such as lymph nodes, some tumors and fluid.

• **Acoustic impedance:** It is the resistance offered by tissues to the movement of particles caused by ultrasonic waves. It is equal to the product of the tissue density and the speed of the ultrasound wave in the tissue. Because of the difference in tissue impedance, US can form images of the part of the body being examined.

Ways used for the exam

Transvaginal way: It has been used preferably in larger species (bovines, buffaloes, and horses. The transducer is introduced towards the bottom of the vagina on one side of the cervix, manipulating the desired organ transrectal with the other hand (preferably ovaries), taking them to the free end of the transducer. It is frequently used in gynecological studies, follicular dynamics (waves of follicular growth) and in follicular aspirations (punctures).

Transrectal way: In the case of cattle, buffaloes and horses, the hand is introduced through the rectum that contains the transducer between the fingers and the desired structure is located (uterus, ovaries, etc.). It is recommended for early diagnosis of pregnancy, as well as sexing, determination of gestational age and fetus viability. In the case of sheep and goats, only the transducer manipulated with the index finger is introduced through the rectum.

Transabdominal way: It is mainly used for the diagnosis of pregnancy in sheep and goats, as well as for the detection of the number of fetuses in these species. This technique is also used in sows and small animals for the diagnosis of pregnancy, as well as for the diagnosis of different genital diseases (e.g. in dogs).

Among the main applications of ultrasonography in reproduction are:

Ultrasonographic morphology of the ovary, ovulation, dynamics of follicular growth, morphology of the corpus luteum, dynamics and morphology of the uterus, anatomopathological diagnoses of the genital tract (pyometra, metritis, salpingitis, hydrosalpinx, etc.).

Early diagnosis of pregnancy with ultrasonography

One of the most widespread applications in the field of reproduction is the early diagnosis of pregnancy in different species (cattle, buffalo, horses, pigs, sheep, and goats, etc.). It is generally accepted that after day 23 in cattle, 15 in horses, 19 in sheep and 25 in goats, it is possible to perform early pregnancy diagnosis with an efficiency close to 100 %.

Transrectal ultrasound examination in cows

In the cow, evacuation of the rectum is not recommended, since the greater flaccidity of its walls often allows air to be introduced, and this complicates correct manipulation and vision of the organs to be studied.

It is advisable to carry out simultaneous manipulation of the transducer and genital tract, positioning them according to the structure that is sought to be studied.

It is very important to keep in mind that, before starting to work with the ultrasound machine, the veterinarian must have a lot of practice in rectal examination by palpation, since both techniques work as a symbiosis, and complement each other to achieve a good result. It is said that in the routine manipulation with the ultrasound machine, "extra hands" and organization are required.

Although ultrasound diagnosis is only two to three weeks earlier than digital rectal examination, it is a faster, more objective technique and allows for more accurate clinical diagnoses (early embryonic death, metritis, pyometra, macerated or mummified fetuses, etc.).

The transducer of choice is the dual frequency transrectal and linear transducer (5-7.5 or 6-8 MHz), since it is very small and can be easily maneuvered, with a good contact surface (7 cm).

Early pregnancy diagnosis in the cow can be made from day 25 post-service. The transrectal ultrasound examination between days 26 and 33 has a sensitivity of 97 % and a specificity of 87 %. At this stage, the embryo measures approximately 1 cm. By day 40, structures such as the head, rump, limbs and umbilical cord can be differentiated.

Other applications of the ultrasound machine

Ultrasonography or ultrasound is a technique through which the evaluation of reproductive events in animals of productive interest can be optimized and improved.

All reproductive processes can be monitored using ultrasound, from the dynamics of follicular waves, the determination of ovulation, the diagnosis of ovarian and uterine diseases, the early detection of pregnancy and the sex of the fetus, as well as early embryonic losses.

It should be used after having very good practice in rectal palpation, performing good training in the handling and care of the equipment, as well as in the interpretation of the images, to achieve the best use of this technology.

This is a very useful tool, both for work in production conditions and for research and teaching work.

Chapter 5

Dysfunctions of the estrous cycle

Content:
Introduction. Postpartum anoestrus. Functional anoestrus. Negative zootechnical factors associated with functional anoestrus. Anoestral cycles. Irregular estrous cycles. Cystic ovarian disease. The repeat breeding cow.

Introduction

Infertility can be a serious problem in livestock farming, especially for highly producing dairy cows. During the postpartum period, cows must have a rapid and favorable involution of the uterus and normal resumption of ovarian activity, followed by accurate detection of estrus with a high conception rate after AI or mating. All of this must occur even if the cow produces a large amount of milk, is in early postpartum and has a negative energy balance. For all those reasons, it's no surprise that reproductive disorders are a common problem. Early diagnosis and appropriate treatment are necessary to achieve and maintain good fertility in the herd.

The reproductive disorders that most affect dairy cows can be divided into the following groups:

I. Cows are not observed in heat.
II. The repeat breeding cows.
III. The intervals of the estrous cycle are irregular.

Postpartum anoestrus

In cattle, an anovulatory period of variable duration normally occurs after calving, because the pituitary gland is not sensitive to the action of GnRH. LH pulses are infrequent, and the amounts of estrogen and progesterone produced by the ovaries are minimal. The length of the calving, first mating or insemination interval varies greatly and depends on the breed, nutritional level, milk yield, season of the year and the calf rearing system.

In herds with a medium nutritional level, most European dairy breed cows have an ICFI of 60-70 days and in crossbreed cows 70-90 days. Zebu cows raised in an extensive management system have an ICFI that ranges between 160-180 days. This long period of postpartum anestrus is typical of beef breed cattle nursing the calf.

Functional anoestrus

Functional anoestrus is the prolongation of postpartum anoestrus, due to uncorrected endogenous overloads (lactation with low nutritional level), which are accentuated after calving, but can also manifest in heifers with delayed puberty.

I use the word "functional" to designate a temporary alterative state, produced by endocrine imbalances in stressful situations, which is susceptible to disappearing quickly and completely. This definition is useful to understand that functional anoestrus is not a disease, but a consequence of inappropriate zootechnical actions.

Zootechnical actions associated with functional anoestrus

Dietary deficiencies are the most important factors that cause ovarian inactivity. In tropical livestock, the supply of nutrients varies considerably between season of the year, in such a way that during the dry season there is a considerable deficit of food to meet the requirements of the animal. The limited supply of energy in the diet influences ovarian function in pre- and postpartum heifers, both by reducing the follicular diameter and by reducing the persistence of the dominant follicle and delaying the start of growth of large follicles.

Prolonged dietary energy restriction results in cessation of estrous cycles in cows and heifers. A reduction of 2.1 mm in the maximum follicular diameter and 50 hours of persistence of the dominant follicle has been observed in two groups of *Bos taurus* heifers fed with different rations and that differed 38 kg in their live weights. Pre-pubertal heifers fed to gain 0.3 kg/d had a smaller follicular diameter than those fed to gain 0.9 kg/d.

The gradual decrease in body mass leading to nutritional anoestrus is accompanied by a gradual decrease in follicular diameter of 0.3 mm in diameter and 6 hours of follicular persistence for every 10 kg of body mass reduction.

Evolution of the ovaries during anoestrus

Postpartum follicular growth patterns vary from animal to animal. Some cows have relatively inactive ovaries, where follicular growth does not exceed a diameter of 10 mm, while others have follicles larger than 10 mm, between 10-15 days after calving. Insufficient LH secretion, caused by nutritional stress, suppresses ovarian functionality. It is important to make a distinction between an anovulatory inactive ovary and an active ovary in which the dominant follicle develops but does not ovulate.

This last case is observed in zebu cattle that breastfeed their young, where follicular waves occur, but ovulation does not, due to the inhibition of the LH surge, because of to the stimulation of breast-feeding.

The variations in ovarian morphology during anoestrus indicate that inactive ovaries reduce their volume due to little or no follicular growth, but the primordial and primary follicles, which constitute the functional unit of the gonads, do not change in size. Therefore, it cannot be said that the small ovaries observed in some zebu cows with functional anoestrus are atrophied ovaries. (See Chap. 4).

Diagnosis

The diagnosis of functional anoestrus is based on clinical symptoms and the comprehensive zootechnical evaluation of the unit. The main symptom is the low frequency of heat observed in the herd, both in cows and heifers of pubertal age.

To carry out the diagnosis effectively, I recommend following the following order:

First. Carry out a study of individual reproductive performance and obtain the reproductive indicators ICFS, CI, anoestrus period, and the total number of open cows. A percentage of 25 to 30 of cattle females with more than 90 days without being detected in heat indicates the existence of anoestrus.

Second. Conduct an examination of the physical condition of the females in the herd. 30 % or more of emaciated cattle females demonstrate that the diet received is below nutritional requirements. In heifers, the weight and age at which they were incorporated into the herd should be investigated and their physical condition verified.

Third. Evaluate the behavior of daily milk production and examine the quantity and quality of food provided to the cows. Dairy cows respond to nutritional stress by reducing the volume of milk produced, along with decreasing body mass. Not only the quantity of food supplied in the ration should be evaluated, but also its quality.

Fourth. Verify, through rectal examination, the functionality of the ovaries and the state of the uterine horns. In functional anoestrus, the uterus is in the pelvic cavity or near the abdominal cavity, the cervix is closed, and the uterine horns are symmetrical and flaccid. The ovaries have a hard-elastic consistency; In others, small follicles can be palpated, and the consistency becomes more elastic.

The unequivocal sign of functional anestrus is the absence of a corpus luteum in the ovaries. At this point I emphasize that complete ovarian functionality is verified solely by the presence or absence of a palpable corpus luteum.

It may happen that, within the group of females reported as functionally anoestric, some appear that have anoestrus caused by other causes: pregnancy, unobserved heat, mummified fetus, pyometra or ovarian hypoplasia. In all these processes, except in ovarian hypoplasia, a CL can be palpated in any of the ovaries, which, with its secretion of progesterone, inhibits ovulation.

Treatment

The treatment of any condition or disease must be directed to the primary cause that produces it. In the case of functional anestrus, interpretive errors of cause and effect have been made that distort the essence of the problem. This has given rise to hormonal therapeutic schemes being used in livestock companies to treat a functional disorder, caused primarily by nutritional stress in livestock. With this procedure, the effect is being combated, but not the cause, which is ultimately the most important. On the other hand, anoestrus is a disorder that affects the entire herd, which entails greater expenses and work. In truth, hormonal treatment will only be justified when some females remain in anoestrus for many days after having recovered their normal body mass.

Below I explain the hormonal treatment schemes that have offered the best results in clinical practice.

Hormonal therapy for the induction of estrus

Numerous therapeutic procedures have been tried for the induction of estrous, including acupuncture, homeopathy, massage of the ovaries and uterus and others, with questionable, inconsistent, and impractical results. The best responses have been obtained with the administration of exogenous stimulating hormones.

Serum gonadotropin (PMSG)

It can be used alone or after previous preparation with progesterone in oil solution.

Technique

Previous preparation with progesterone is carried out by injecting 50 mg of progesterone via IM three times with 48 hour intervals. This is done so that progesterone acts by reducing the threshold of response to serum chorionic gonadotropin. Then after 48 hours the last treatment, 500 to 600 IU of PMSG are injected IM. 65 to 70 % of treated females should present complete heat syndrome within 24 to 36 hours following treatment. Sometimes 10-15 % of treated females have an ovarian response, but do not show psychological signs of heat. For this reason, it is also indicated to inseminate those that are not in heat, 24 and 36 hours after the last treatment.

Human chorionic gonadotropin or hCG

Technique

It can be used in combination with PMSG to ensure ovulation. The required dose for heifers is 1,200 IU and 1,500 IU in cows, via IM. In practice, hCG is not used to induce heat, due to its high cost.

Estradiol benzoate (BE)

Technique

With a dose of 0.5 mg via IM, heat can be induced in the cow within 12 to 36 hours after treatment. In animals with good body condition, 90 % heat can be reached, with 30 % ovulation. For this reason, it is recommended to inseminate treated females from the second spontaneous heat.

Anoestral cycles

The anoestral cycle is one in which the cow has normal ovarian functionality, but there is an absence or decrease in external signs of heat; That is, there is ovulation, but there is no expressiveness of the heat syndrome. This type of silent heat usually appears in the first heats after calving, especially in dairy breed cows that have been stabled for some time.

Symptoms and diagnosis

Silent heat and postpartum anoestrus can be confused since the female does not express the external symptoms of heat. An important element is that silent heat usually occurs in the first heats of stabled dairy cows. That is, between 25 to 45 days postpartum. The definitive diagnosis will be based on rectal examination to discover the presence of a cyclic corpus luteum in one of its ovaries

But the main difficulty is in determining whether it is short heat or undetected heat due to poor observation. In tropical livestock, diagnostic errors can be made by confusing functional anestrus with silent heat. This occurs when the type of animal, or the conditions of exploitation and management, are not considered.

On the other hand, most veterinary technicians and inseminating technicians do not have skills in palpating the ovaries or recognizing the corpora lutea.

I emphasize that the incidence of silent heat in the conditions of exploitation that prevails in extensive breeding is very unlikely, since prolonged stabling of animals is not practiced there.

Estrous cycles with irregular intervals

The normal length of the estrous cycle is 18-24 days. Shorter or longer estrous intervals are considered abnormal during the reproductive period. Intervals of 6 to 9 weeks are very common in flocks with poor heat detection. Cystic ovarian disease and embryonic mortality are the most important causal agents of irregular estrous cycles. Short sexual cycles in the early postpartum period are not considered abnormal.

Cystic ovarian disease

Ovarian cysts are defined as large fluid-filled structures in one or both ovaries, which persist for more than 40 days postpartum and are accompanied by abnormal behavior of the sexual cycle (estrus with irregular intervals, hyperestrus or anestrus).

Etiopathogenesis

There is evidence that indicates a hereditary predisposition to ovarian cysts in certain pedigree lines of dairy cows. The incidence of cysts is also higher in high milk producing cows aged 5-6 years and 30-45 days postpartum. This coincides with the maximum stress induced by milk secretion. It is hypothesized that lactation stress interferes with the release of LH.

Some puerperal problems such as retained placenta, milk fever and metritis have been associated with an increase in ovarian cysts. In the case of metritis, endo and exotoxins induce high levels of cortisol that can interfere with the preovulatory LH wave.

Clinically, two types of cysts are recognized: follicular and luteal.

Follicular cysts

These develop from Graafian follicles that have failed to ovulate (indehiscent) and that enlarge considerably when filled with fluid (< 2.5 cm in diameter). I must warn that a large proportion of follicular cysts of this size can be found in the ovaries of dairy cows during the puerperal period as a normal phase in the physiological process of reestablishing ovarian activity. Only those that persist beyond 40 days postpartum can be considered true cysts and require some treatment.

On rectal examination, the cyst is palpated as a fluctuating lump protruding from the ovary, but sometimes the gonad turns into a smooth-surfaced cystic sac the size of a pigeon or chicken egg.

If the cyst has a very thin wall, it ruptures easily when palpated. Those with thicker walls are turgid and resistant to palpation. (Fig. 5-1).

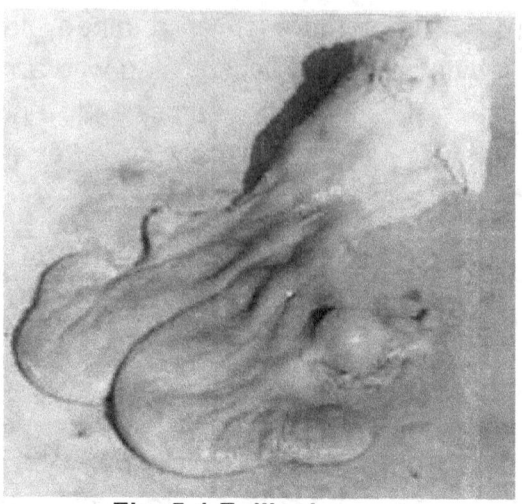

Fig. 5-1 Follicular cyst

Diagnosis

It is important to locate yourself in the type of animal that makes up the herd. When it comes to cows with medium to low milk yield, the probability of this disorder appearing is low.

The most striking symptom of tight-walled follicular cysts is hyperestronism. The cow shows signs of intense heat that lasts for several days. On rectal palpation, one or more cysts may be found, in one or both ovaries.

The hyperestronism of cystic ovarian disease must be differentiated from that of nymphomania, which is very rare and has an extraovarian (adrenal gland) origin.

The flaccid wall follicular cyst, on the other hand, presents with anoestrus. On rectal palpation, the uterus shows unequivocal signs of anoestrus: closed neck, flaccid horns.

In the ovaries you can find one or more follicular cysts with very thin walls and no turgor, like a balloon partially filled with water. This type of cyst often ruptures just by palpating it.

Luteal cysts

It forms from a developed corpus luteum that, for unknown reasons, forms a cavity within the luteal tissue and fills with fluid causing it to grow two to three times its normal size. The CL cyst produces progesterone and affects the length of the estrous cycle by inhibiting estrus.

I must say that, in my work as a Professor of Veterinary Gynecology for five decades, I found, in many cases, normal corpora lutea, but cavitaries filled with a clear and transparent liquid, in the ovaries of cows from different slaughterhouses. I clarify that the cavity observed was small. This fact has also been observed through ovarian ultrasound performed on different cows, including pregnant cows.

Differential diagnosis

The follicular cyst has a thin wall and is fluctuant on palpation, while the luteal cyst has a thicker layer of luteal tissue on the wall of the cyst, making it more consistent under pressure. The follicular cyst tends to be multiple, but not the luteal cyst. Clinically, follicular cysts with tight walls tend to produce hyperestrus, but many of them present with anestrus. Luteal cysts are less common and are associated with anestrus; However, differentiation between both cysts based on sexual behavior is not possible since some follicular cysts with flaccid walls also present with anoestrus.

The luteal cyst has the peculiarity that it is unique and is much less common. On rectal examination, the cyst is palpated as a rounded formation four or more cm in diameter; It has a more compact consistency than the follicular cyst due to the greater thickness of its wall, but some fluctuation of the liquid it contains can be noted. Manual rupture of this cyst is more difficult and can cause injury to the ovarian tissue.

Treatment

GnRH administration is the treatment of choice. This hormone induces luteinization of follicular cysts. Depending on the type of cyst and possibility of GnRH dosage, some follicular cysts may be induced to rupture. 60-80 % of cows show heat between 18 and 23 days after the injection of 250 mcg of GnRH, in a dose of 5 ml via IM.

Cows that have not come into heat within 25 days of treatment with GnRH or hCG should be checked and re-treated if necessary.

The administration of 3,000 IU of hCG intravenously is another possibility. A combination of 3,000 IU of hCG and 125 mg of progesterone, simultaneously by slow intravenous route, has been effective for the treatment of follicular cysts that present with hyperestronism.

The oldest and least expensive treatment is manual rupture of the follicular cyst. Rectally, the meso-ovary is fixed between the index and middle fingers and moderate pressure is applied to the cyst, against the palm of the hand, until it bursts. This pressure should be done with the fingertips to avoid trauma.

The potential danger of trauma to the ovary is that it causes hemorrhage with subsequent local adhesions, this should not be ruled out, but manual disruption is harmless, if done correctly. This method must be weighed against the cost of hormone therapy. It has been reported 37 % to 63 % of recoveries; however, the cyst can recur. When excessive force is required to rupture the cyst, especially thick-walled luteal cysts, manual rupture should not be insisted upon.

The repeat breeding cow (RB)

Definition

Repeat breeding is infertility of variable duration, which appears in cyclical cows, in which their genital apparatus is apparently normal and which, having been inseminated with fertile semen, do not conceive after at least three successive services.

Due to the multiple causes that produce it and the difficulties in identifying them, some Anglo-Saxon authors designate it as Sterility sine materia or *Causa ignota*.

Causes of repeat breeding

The causes of RB can be of three types: biological, environmental, and biotechnological. Most of them can be grouped into failure of ovulation, including fractional estrus, impossibility of encounter between zoosperms and eggs after ovulation due to anatomical anomalies, subclinical genital infections, inadequate gametic transport, asynchrony between insemination and ovulation, fertilization failure, implantation failure and abortion. As can be seen, it is almost impossible to pinpoint the causes of conception failure in individual cases.

Biological and environmental causes

Under the conditions of Cuban tropical livestock farming, repetition of services was focused on Holstein breed herds, which was the most widespread dairy breed in the country. In addition to the genetic factor, high milk production and dysfunction of the corpus luteum caused by RS due to insufficient production of progesterone influence this breed.

In a study carried out in Sancti Spiritus, we were able to verify that 54 % of repeater cows showed abnormal serum progesterone profiles. None of the 35 cows with luteal dysfunction conceived, while 25 of 30 cows with normal progesterone profiles became pregnant. It is very likely that the hormonal dysfunction was associated with the environmental heat stress that the Holstein cows suffered during most of the year.

It is noteworthy that Holstein heifers were not affected by RS syndrome and maintained a fertility potential like that of crossbred heifers. From which it is deduced that dairy production played an important role in the genesis of RS of this breed.

Infectious causes

In some texts and scientific articles, it is still stated that latent subclinical infections caused by non-specific germs harm the gametes and even the embryo itself. They even recommend administering antibiotic solutions intrauterine, 24 hours after A.I. However, considering current knowledge these statements are inconsistent.

Our group was able to verify that the bacteriological flora of the vagina, cervix, and uterus of cows with repeated services is identical to that of fertile cows.

Furthermore, the histopathological studies that we carried out on sections of uteri from repeater cows did not reveal any alterations of any kind, even in those that presented purulent and muco-purulent secretions in the cervico-vaginal duct. (See Charter 6).

According to these results, the subclinical form of chronic catarrhal endometritis that many authors have postulated as causing infertility or infertility has no scientific support.

Biotechnological factors

It can be stated that biotechnological factors are responsible for most RS cases that occur in dairy cows in the country. These factors include errors in the application of the A.I. technique, poor semen conservation, inseminating at inappropriate times of heat, or without being in heat, inseminating cows during the postpartum period, and others.

Symptoms and pathogenesis

The most expressive symptom is infertility of variable duration. The intervals between mattings or inseminations can have the duration of a normal cycle of 18-21 days, when fertilization does not occur, but generally tend to be longer than 24 days if embryonic mortality (EM) has occurred. This occurs during the first two phases of zygote development: during the ovular period and during the embryonic period. The degeneration of the zygote represents the first stage of early ME and in which the division of the blastomeres occurs irregularly.

EM during organogenesis develops in the following times: reabsorption of embryonic fluid, decomposition of the embryo and decomposition of fetal membranes. In the cow, the embryo can disappear while the embryonic envelopes and the corpus luteum remain, which results in a prolonged anestrus because of an occupied uterus.

In a study carried out to determine the repetitiveness of RB in Holstein and Siboney cows, we found that most cows had repetition of services only once in their reproductive life. The 9.5 % of Holsteins and 5.3 % of Siboney had it three times in their entire lives.

I have personally observed Holstein cows that have required up to ten services per conception and only one after that. These facts demonstrate that RB is not a condition that affects a specific animal, but rather occurs in any predisposed animal.

How repeat breeding is diagnosed and treated

The causes of RB do not affect all herds or all breeds equally. Therefore, the diagnosis depends on the type of animal considered.

Dairy cows

This type of cattle, which is characterized by its high milk yield, has a recognized predisposition to show repetitions of three or more services.

For the clinician, it is important to know if the repetitions are due to infertility or infertility. When there are failures in fertilization, the interval between inseminations is 18-21 days and does not alter the length of the normal cycle.

This allows us to reason that the causes that are influencing are biotechnological in nature and to act accordingly.

The inability of the zygote to continue growing and developing until it becomes a full-term fetus constitutes infertility.

When the death of the embryo occurs early, the intervals between inseminations tend to exceed 24 days, sometimes 40-45 days or more.

Beef cows and their crossbreeds

In cows of this type, the frequency of RB is relatively low and when it occurs it is due to technical errors of the A.I. or poor reproductive management.

How to reduce RB in dairy cattle

A wide variety of hormonal treatments have been tested with the purpose of reducing the incidence of SR and shortening the PI; among them GnRH, progesterone, hCG and recombinant interferon α-1 (rIFN-α). These treatments, in addition to being expensive, have not had the expected effectiveness.

Since environmental heat stress is the causal agent that most affects RB in tropical herds, the alternative to reduce its presence is to improve the microclimate where the animals live and ensure a balanced diet throughout the year. It is also necessary to take zootechnical measures that promote the development of reproductive physiological processes and avoid stressful states before and after A.I. In many cases it is enough to apply corrective measures in the reproductive management of the herd or in the A.I. technique. as a whole.

The veterinarian or zootechnician must assess the reproductive situation from a comprehensive point of view, involving biological, environmental, and biotechnological factors and start with the latter, which is more easily detectable and measurable.

Chapter 6

Inflammatory processes of the genital tract

Content:
Defense mechanism of the uterus. Pathophysiology of the puerperium. Metritis. Subacute endometritis. Pyometra. Non-inflammatory vaginal leucorrhea and its clinical significance. Cervicitis. Cervical stenosis. Vaginitis. Vulvitis and vulvar craurosis.

Introduction

Normally the uterus is protected from the external environment by the vulva, the vestibular sphincter, and the cervix. Other effective defensive mechanisms also participate, such as hormonal (estrogen, oxytocin), enzymes, and the reticuloendothelial system, which allow fertilization, development, and birth of the fetus, without the need for human intervention. However, because of genetic selection, dairy cows, particularly high-yielding ones, have become more vulnerable to the conditions of the external environment and sometimes their natural defensive mechanisms fail, especially after calving.

The lack of hygiene in childbirth care, and traumatic obstetric procedures, predispose cows to suffer from uterine infections, which are more frequent in dairy breeds, since milk production creates a state of lower resistance.

This chapter addresses the inflammatory processes of the genital tract that have had the greatest impact on the conditions of the tropical ecosystem.

Defense mechanism of the uterus

The cow's uterus is an organ that is histologically prepared against insults that may affect it. It has a histological structure with a high power of regeneration and mobilization of defensive elements from the reticuloendothelial system, local self-purification mechanisms, all associated with the endocrine balance, represented, above all, by the secretions of oxytocin, PGF2α and estrogens. Under the influence of estrogen, the uterus has a high degree of antimicrobial activity, making it highly resistant to infections during the estrogenic phase.

The production of local antibodies and phagocytosis via opsonins are defense mechanisms that limit the duration of uterine infections. Cytokines also play important roles as autocrine and paracrine regulators, as well as interferon gamma, in the reproductive tract.

The normal endometrium can mount a local response to pathogen invasion and maintaining it in a sterile environment.

For the recognition of the immune response, it is necessary that cells are present for the recognition of the antigen and that immuno-regulatory lymphocytes and macrophages are present. Endometrial lymphocytes are intra-epithelial lymphocytes with functional characteristics like those of the intestine. Progesterone inhibits the proliferation of endometrial lymphocytes and myometrial contractility.

Pathophysiology of puerperium

The mechanism responsible for the elimination of germs from the uterus and the death of migrating leukocytes is phagocytosis, helped by the activity of uterine contractions, the elimination of caruncular tissue, resorption, and expulsion of contaminated lochia. The normal flora acts as the host's primary defense by competition.

Failures in the defense mechanism can be an important factor in the development of uterine infections in cattle and in the failure of therapeutic agents to eliminate these infections. Trauma to the genital tract from placental extraction or other obstetric procedures also depresses phagocytosis.

Some antimicrobial drugs and disinfectants infused into the uterus decrease the uterine defense mechanism and irritate and strip the endometrium.

Uterine involution

Uterine involution begins with the reduction in the size of the organ due to vasoconstriction and contractions of the myometrium. During the first 10 days, involution is relatively slow; From day 10 to 14 there is a marked increase in tone and reduction in the size of the uterus.

After 15 days the uterus can be completely palpated and after 20-30 days it has reached its normal size. The cervix involutes more slowly and returns to normal after 40-50 days postpartum.

Lochia

The day after childbirth the uterus contains approximately 1.5 liters, after the 8th day 0.5 liters; This fluid is serous-bloody, later it becomes darker, with cellular debris and the smell of fresh meat. After a week, the lochia acquires a pastier, pus-like consistency.

This material can be confused with purulent discharges. After 12-14 days the lochia is denser, scarcer and chocolate colored. After 15-18 days they are crystalline, like estrous mucus and then they disappear almost completely. Clinical evidence of uncomplicated progress of uterine involution is the lack of secretions and the absence of odor.

Retained placenta (RP)

Placental expulsion is the technical term that exists to designate the detachment and elimination of the secundines or fetal membranes. In the cow, the placenta is normally expelled within 6-8 hours after calving.

It is considered that there is retained placenta when the secundines have not been eliminated within 24 hours postpartum. The incidence of placental retention varies from 4 to 16 % but can be much higher in problem dairy herds.

Etiology and lesions

Retained placenta can be influenced by multiple factors, including genetic, nutritional, immunological, infectious, and mechanical. All of them can alter the mechanism of detachment of the chorionic villi slightly attached to the cotyledons.

Fetal membranes and their fluids, retained in the uterus, are an excellent breeding ground for the development of saprophytic bacteria or bacteria introduced from the outside during childbirth.

More than 30 different species of bacteria have been identified in the lumen of the uterus during the puerperium, the most frequent being: *Actinomyces pyogenes, Escherichia coli, streptococci,* and *staphylococci.*

Coliforms and streptococci are enterobacteria that contaminate, probably non-pathogenic, the genital tract.

Coliforms are frequently isolated in the early puerperium, but to a lesser extent in retained placenta and metritis. In research carried out by our group, we verified that the bacteriological flora found in the vagina and uterus of recently calved, healthy empty cows with repeated services, corresponded to the germs classified as facultative pathogens and apathogenic. The most isolated were *E. coli, Micrococus aureus, Micrococus albus, streptococci sp, Seudomona aureuginosa.* However, *A. pyogenes* had a low incidence.

Under tropical livestock farming conditions, the factors that most influence the appearance of RP are malnutrition during pregnancy and disorders associated with parturition (dystocic births, laborious births), which tend to produce secondary uterine hypotonia or atony due to myometrial depletion. Laborious calvings are more common in heifers and Holstein cows because they give birth to large calves.

Treatment

Medications administered intrauterine postpartum are ineffective due to the nature of the puerperal intrauterine environment.

On the other hand, drugs that increase uterine motility (oxytocin, ergonovine) have been ineffective for the expulsion of fetal membranes.

When cows have eutocic or normal births and are in good body condition, RP are resolved by the defensive system of the uterus and do not require treatment. However, in all cases, the professional must be alert to changes in the animal's behavior and local symptoms, especially the production of dark and fetid lochia.

If the fetal membranes hang from the vulva, their detachment can be assisted mechanically by wrapping the membranes around a wooden rod and pulling them down with some pressure. If the membranes do not come off by this procedure, it is better not to force them and let them necrotize and come off on their own, within 7-10 days postpartum. The evacuation of lochia can also be helped by gentle compression of the uterus through the rectum.

The most convenient thing is to apply the conservative method, which consists of letting the process evolve without local intervention. Vaginal and intrauterine manipulation and attempts to manually separate the fetal membranes are contraindicated, since this operation produces trauma and there is a danger of exacerbating latent vaginal and uterine inflammatory processes, due to depression of uterine phagocytosis.

The objective of treatment must be to prevent the adverse effects of toxemic metritis, associated with RP. Therefore, attention must be directed to those cows with RP that show signs of inappetence, lassitude, fever (40-41°C), reduced milk secretion, or mastitis, concomitant with blackish, abundant, and foul-smelling lochial secretions. With this clinical picture, the most indicated is to apply immediate parenteral treatment with broad-spectrum antibiotics since there is a risk of death due to toxemia or bacteremia. When the affected cow falter and falls into a state of prostration, the prognosis is very serious, and it has very little chance of survival.

Acute inflammation of uterus

Depending on the course and severity of the process, acute inflammation of the uterus can present in two clinical forms, toxemic metritis, and acute metritis.

Acute metritis

Metritis is the acute and sometimes over-acute inflammatory process that affects the three layers that make up the uterus, which are the perimetrium, the outermost layer, the mesometrium or middle layer, formed by the stroma and the myometrium, and the endometrium, the inner layer, formed by the uterine mucosa with its glands.

This disorder occurs in the first days after childbirth and, with some exceptions, is associated with retained placenta. It usually appears after dystocic births in which obstetric maneuvers have been performed, with injuries to the soft birth canal, which cause uterine hypotony.

The microorganisms usually most involved in acute metritis are *Actinomises pyogenes, group C streptococci, hemolytic staphylococci*, Gram-anaerobic bacteria, coliform agents and rarely clostridium. The germs and their toxins are absorbed into the general circulation, causing septicemia, toxemia and sometimes pyemia, that is, toxiinfection. There may be a pathogenic synergism between *A. pyogenes* and *F. necrophorum*, to cause an increase in the severity of postpartum uterine infections, with the subsequent altering effect on the return to estrus and conception. Cows that do not fully recover from *A. pyogenes* infection within 40-50 days postpartum tend to develop subacute mucopurulent endometritis or pyometra.

Symptoms

Inflammation of the uterus can present as severe toxemic metritis, the clinical signs of which appear one to ten days after delivery and last two to six days.

A watery, reddish, or chocolatey, extremely fetid vulvar discharge is characteristic, accompanied by uterine inertia and fever of up to 41°C during the first phase of the disease, up to a subnormal temperature, in animals close to death.

In sepsis, symptoms of general depression, anorexia, rapid and weak pulse (80-120 beats/min) and tachypnea appear. Ruminal paresis occurs with the deposition of hard or liquid, black, greasy, foul-smelling feces. There is a marked drop in milk production, and rapid weight loss.

On rectal examination, the uterus appears atonic and with thinned walls, so palpation should be performed gently. Complications are frequent, and peritonitis may occur due to the spread of the infection and acute laminitis that makes the animal unable to stand and remain standing.

The prognosis is guarded to poor unless treatment is started before the uterus is severely damaged. It tends to become more severe when the response to treatment fails and complications such as mastitis, laminitis and pneumonia persist.

Treatment

It should be aimed at overcoming the effects of sepsis and toxemia as soon as possible. Administer IM, in doses of 20,000-25,000 IU/kg, penicillin G sodium, combined with the same dose of procaine penicillin, every 12 hours.

As symptomatic treatment, an antihistamine such as pyranisamine or Urtimine will be administered, in a dose of 1 mg/kg of weight. Systemic treatment will be continued for 3-4 days until the general condition improves and the febrile syndrome subsides.

Drainage of uterine contents rectally may be advantageous but must be performed gently and carefully since manipulation of the puerperal uterus may result in bacteremia.

If the general condition of the animal is very affected, with lameness and danger of death, it is best to use intravascular injections of novocaine, a simpler form of systemic neural blockade, which is used in pathogenic therapy.

To do this, a warm solution of 0.25 % novocaine or lidocaine, diluted in an isotonic NaCl solution, is injected into the cow's jugular vein at a dose of 0.5 ml/kg. The injections are repeated for several days. In the first three treatments it should be combined with antibiotics and then every two days without antibiotics. For example, one gram of Streptomycin with 3 million IU of Penicillin dissolved in a volume of 150 ml of a 0.25 % novocaine or lidocaine solution, during the first three days and then the same novocaine solution in the same dose every other day, twice.

A more effective alternative for these cases is aorta puncture. 100 ml of a 1% novocaine or lidocaine solution is prepared and 3 million IU of Penicillin or three grams of oxytetracycline are added and slowly perfused into the abdominal aorta artery. The dose is repeated on the 2nd or 3rd day.

This treatment has the drawback that it requires a special 18 cm long needle, with a mandrel, to be able to reach and penetrate the artery and adequate mastery of the technique. For more details, see Pathogenic Therapy in the book by Plajotin (1982).

Acute suppurative metritis

Occurs during the first weeks of the puerperium. Unlike toxemic metritis, the general condition of the animal is not affected. The most obvious external symptom is mucopurulent brown or gray vulvar discharge, sometimes fetid. Later, it is common for a creamy yellow or gray discharge from the uterus to adhere only to the tail and to the surroundings of the vulva.

On rectal examination, a large, thickened, and hard uterus can be seen, indicating delayed involution. Vaginal examination reveals a relaxed, dilated, hyperemic neck and a mucopurulent secretion emanating from its lumen.

Treatment

It is very common for acute suppurative metritis to be controlled by the defensive mechanisms of the uterus and to remit without the need for treatment; other times they are attenuated and pass into the subacute stage. When they are severe and with an appreciable delay in the uterine involution process, intravenous or intra-arterial treatment is required, as described for toxemic metritis.

Subacute and chronic endometritis

In this process, only the uterine mucosa or endometrium is affected and most of them are the consequence of acute suppurative metritis or uncured vaginltis.

Symptoms and injuries

Clinical symptoms appear after three weeks postpartum with mucopurulent discharges that are noted when cows lie down to ruminate or when their vagina is examined with a speculum. Subacute suppurative endometritis can also be suspected when muco-purulent secretions, abundant, mixed with cervico-vaginal mucus, are observed during heat or at the time of being inseminated. The estrous cycle usually has a normal duration, but conception failures occur due to early embryonic mortality, which leads to repetitions of services.

Endometritis produces purulent exudates and peri-glandular fibrosis with leukocyte infiltration and subsequent glandular degeneration that modify the uterine environment and prevent nidation. On rectal examination, an insufficiently involuted uterus can be palpated, recognizable by being enlarged, hard to the touch, and with thick walls of a pasty consistency. Upon vaginoscopic examination, the cervix may be hyperemic, enlarged, and mucopurulent or purulent exudates are observed in greater or lesser amounts.

Diagnosis

The clinical diagnosis is based on the anamnesis, mainly what happened in the recent postpartum period and on the external and internal clinical symptoms. At this point I emphasize that every inflammatory process evolves according to the known cardinal signs of inflammation, which alter the affected organ with intensity. If there are no observable clinical signs, inflammation cannot be diagnosed.

As I will demonstrate later, the sole presence of mucopurulent or purulent secretions in the vagina does not justify the diagnosis of subacute endometritis, as has been done until now.

Treatment

Due to the confusion that exists regarding the diagnosis of subacute endometritis and the overvaluation that has been made of the discharge of mucopurulent secretions from the vagina, the treatment of this process is one of the most abundant and varied that has been applied to disease in many countries with the particularity that all of them seemed to be effective.

Most authors agree that antibiotics and other products lose their effectiveness when they are infused into inflamed uterine horns that contain exudates. However, they continue to recommend the intrauterine route for the treatment of subacute endometritis.

When we studied the bacteriological flora of exudates from cows with subacute endometritis, we were able to verify that a high percentage of them were negative to the microbiological examination. This means that, in these processes, the causal agent was attenuated or absent. For this reason, the most rational thing is to get the uterus to reactivate its depressed defensive system and regeneration of the endometrium occurs through natural mechanisms. It should not be overlooked that cows that calve in extensive breeding have a low incidence of uterine inflammation despite not receiving medical care.

The reactivation of the defensive system of the uterus can be achieved depending on the presence or absence of CL in its ovaries. If CL is present in an ovary, IM injection of a PG analogue, at standard luteolytic doses, is indicated. If there is anestrus without CL, heat should be induced with synthetic estrogens. In both cases, what is sought is for the uterus to return to the follicular or estrogenic phase.

Remember that estrogens have uterotonic and mobilizing activity of antibodies and defensive cells of the local reticuloendothelial system.

If the uterine horns have not involuted sufficiently and contain many exudates, intrauterine perfusion of a 1-2 % Lugol's solution is also justified, immediately after the female has come into heat.

Lugol exerts a light irritating action on the endometrium, with hyperemia which activates the local defensive system.

After 30 days, the therapeutic effectiveness of the medications should be checked through a rectal examination. If clinical symptoms have subsided, cows can return to A.I. service. or natural mating.

Pyometra

From a pathological point of view, pyometra is a chronic suppurative endometritis characterized by the progressive accumulation of purulent exudate within the uterine cavity. Clinically, it presents with anestrus due to the persistence of a corpus luteum in the ovary, because of an occupied uterus. In general, the incidence of pyometra in cattle is low.

It has the same etiology as the subacute inflammatory processes described previously; but it also occurs, occasionally, as consequences of death and subsequent fetal maceration in cases of trichomoniasis.

Two clinical forms of pyometra are recognized: open and closed.

Symptoms

The main one is the anestrus. The cow behaves as if she were pregnant. In closed pyometra the animal becomes thinner, and the skin becomes rough, with the hair standing on end. In open pyometra, the cervical canal is open and allows variable amounts of purulent exudates to escape to the outside, observable when the animal lies down. In closed pyometra there is no expulsion of exudates.

Diagnosis

It is based on the anamnesis and external and internal symptomatology. Prolonged anestrus, the expulsion of purulent secretions when lying down, the presence of a persistent CL in one of the ovaries and the absence of a fetus in a distended uterus with thin walls and the failure to observe arterial thrills serve to confirm the diagnosis.

Treatment

If the pyometra is of small volume and of short duration, some benefit can be obtained by injecting a PGF2α analogue IM, for example 50 mg of cloprostenol, so that heat occurs and the opening of the cervix leads to the evacuation of pus. intrauterine.

The pus evacuation effect with this treatment reaches 90 %, if the corpus luteum is present and occurs around 24 hours after the injection. Some cows may need several treatments at intervals of 10 to 14 days to evacuate the pus.

If there is no persistent CL or it is not detected in the ovaries, an attempt can be made to eliminate the pus with an injection of 20-30 mg of Diethylethylbestrol or one milligram of Estradiol Benzoate via IM, to promote uterine contractility.

After total or partial evacuation of the exudate is achieved, perfuse 250-500 ml of 1-2 % Lugol solution into the uterus. After two weeks, evaluate the effect of the treatment and repeat the infusion with Lugol, if necessary.

If the pyometra is voluminous and long-lasting, the degenerative damage to the endometrium is so profound that its regeneration is impossible and the animal will not recover its fertility.

In this case, the treatment described above is applied, so that it evacuates the purulent contents of the uterus and reaches a good nutritional state, and then it is sent to the slaughterhouse.

The false vaginal suppurative exudates in cattle and its clinical significance

The term leucorrhea comes from the Greek "leucos, white and rhea, flow or fluid": whitish discharge from the female genital tract. Technically leucorrhea is an exudate. This is composed of cellular and humoral substances, which accumulate around inflammation. The migration of cellular and humoral substances into an area of inflammation is known as exudation.

The exudate consists of five components:

1- The irritant

2- Cells from the injured tissue

3- Leukocytes

4- Plasma constituents (water, proteins, fibrin, and antibodies)

5- Erythrocytes

The presence of mucopurulent and purulent secretions in the vagina and uterus has always been associated with subacute and chronic inflammatory processes in these organs. In almost all Veterinary Gynecology books, three degrees of endometritis are described in correspondence with the predominance of the type of secretion: catarrhal, purulent catarrhal and purulent.

In a doctoral thesis carried out in Cuba, vaginal exudates were characterized depending on the ways in which the pus was distributed, in the form of stretch marks, flocs, and the diagnosis of different degrees of chronic endometritis in cows was attributed to these findings.

In a study carried out in 1975, because of the work of the National Reproduction Brigade, a finding of 25 % of cows with chronic endometritis was reported. Some scientists from the Animal Improvement Research Center reported similar findings in the province of Havana in 1980.

In the exercise of gynecological practice for five decades, in research work and in the review of thousands of genital organs of cows and heifers from slaughterhouses for teaching practices, I was struck by the presence of mucopurulent and purulent secretions in the vagina of heifers and cows in different stages of the estrous cycle, without macroscopic lesions or signs that denote the presence of inflammatory lesions of the vagina or uterine horns.

These observations motivated me to demonstrate the hypothesis that the presence of collections of vaginal suppurative exudates (leukorrhea) was not always the product of inflammatory or infectious processes of the vagina or uterus.

After numerous observations we found a frequency of collections of suppurative exudates in 12 % of heifers and 20 % in cows. Only 6.3 % of the histological preparations of vaginas and 8.8 % of those of the uterus showed mild microscopic lesions.

The pH of the vaginal secretions was 6.9 and no differences were found in the electrophoretic spectrum of the protein molecules or nucleic acids contained in the leukorrheic and non-leukorrheic samples. No inflammatory cells were found in any of the stained smears.

It was found that the bacterial and fungal species isolated from the mucosa of vaginas and uterine horns of cows without and with mucopurulent and purulent secretions were practically the same, in presence and frequency, as the germs considered facultative pathogens (See Table 6-2).

Enterobacteriaceae represented close to 50 % of the isolates. However, A. *pyogenes*, S. *viridans*, S. *epidermidis* and S. *aureus* (which are the bacterial agents considered pyogenic) were present in only 25 % of the isolates.

Conception rates at first service obtained in 150 virgin heifers and 474 cows without and with leucorrhea were 79.8 % vs 81.8 % and 75.0 % vs 76.0 % for heifers and cows respectively.

These results allowed us to conclude that the leukorrheal secretions observed are not exudates but modified mucous secretions that do not have an inflammatory or infectious origin.

Table 6-2 Comparative microbiological examination

Microorganism	Without false exudates				With exudates			
	Vagina		Uterus		Vagina		Uterus	
	n	%	n	%	n	%	n	%
Escherichia coli	30	25,0	32	26,6	6	15,0	3	16,6
E. colivar. hemolítica	6	5,0	12	13,3	8	20,0	3	12,5
Klebsiella aerogenes	6	5,0	3	20,0	2	5,0	2	8,3
Protes vulgaris	3	2,5	-	-	-	-	-	-
Shigell adysenteriae	6	5,0	18	26,6	2	5,0	2	8,3
Haffnia sp.	-	-	-	-	3	7,5	4	16,6
Streptococcus sp.	12	10,0	-	-	-	-	-	-
Streptococcus αhemolitico	8	7,7	-	-	-	-	-	-
Streptococcus viridans	-	-	-	-	6	15,0	2	8,3
Streptococcus durans	-	-	-	-	2	5,0	-	-
Streptococcus faecalis	-	-	-	-	3	7,5	2	8,3
Staphylococcus epidermidis	24	20,5	-	-	4	10,0	3	12,5
Staphylococcus aureus	18	15,4	-	-	1	2,5	2	8,3
Staphylococcus citreus	-	-	-	-	3	7,5	2	8,3
Pasteurella hemolitica	6	5,0	12	13,3	-	-	-	-
Arcanobacterium pyogenes	3	2,5	6	6,6	4	10,0	1	4,1
Pseudomonas aeruginosa	4	4,0	-	-	-	-	-	-
Sarcina lutea	18	15,4	-	-	2	5,0	-	-
Rhizopusrhiz odifurmis	18	15,0	-	-	2	5,0	-	-
Candida albicans	9	8,0	-	-	3	7,5	-	-
Aspergillus fumigatus	6	5,0	-	-	-	-	-	-
Mucorr acemosus	6	5,0	-	-	-	-	-	-

Since the existence of false suppurative vaginal exudates is not reported in the literature consulted at the national and international level, the results obtained are a scientific discovery that questions the high incidence of subacute and chronic endometritis reported in Cuba by some researchers and allows understand the reason for the effectiveness of the multiple and sometimes disconcerting therapeutic means used to treat "*subacute and chronic endometritis*".

Diagnostic significance of vaginal exudates

The presence of mucopurulent or purulent pseudo-exudates, more or less abundant in the vagina of heifers or cows, in any period of the estrous cycle or in a state of pregnancy, not accompanied by clinical signs of inflammation, (hyperemia, edema, erosions of the mucosa) should be considered as false vaginal suppurative exudates, which are temporary and do not affect the fertility or health of the females that present it.

Cervicitis

The cervix is inappropriately considered, by some authors, as the mirror of the womb. An inflamed neck, with purulent exudates, can indicate the existence of endometritis or metritis, but it can also coexist with vaginitis. Frequently, cervical injuries are of traumatic origin, occurring during childbirth. Cervicitis is rarely primary or idiopathic.

On vaginal examination, the cervix appears hyperemic and somewhat edematous, sometimes obstructed by a purulent mass. If vaginitis is present, the mucosa is hyperemic, congested, eroded, with collections of muco-purulent or purulent exudates.

Diagnosis and treatment

After vaginoscopy, the condition of the uterine horns should be checked rectally. Consider the existence of a recent birth and signs of inflammation of the uterine horns. If there is no palpable structural modification of the horns, chronic metritis should be ruled out.

In case of cervico-vaginitis, the treatment to follow is that indicated for vaginitis. If there is concomitant metritis, treatment for chronic metritis should be applied.

Cervical stenosis

Non-congenital cervical canal stenosis and obstruction are very rare in cattle. In chapter 4, we explained that neither the enlargement nor the U or S shaped cervical curve of *Bos taurus indicus* cows or their crossbreeds affect the permeability of the cervical lumen.

Vaginitis or colpitis

Inflammations of the vagina, due to their course, can be acute or subacute and due to their origin, primary or secondary.

Primary acute vaginitis

Occurs because of laborious births, large fetuses, inadequate traction of the calf in dystocic births, which lead to tears and wounds in the mucosa of the vagina and cervix.

This traumatic postpartum vaginitis is generally resolved by the organ's self-defense systems unless the lesions are very extensive.

Subacute primary vaginitis

Can be due to non-specific infections coming from the bacteriological and fungal flora of the vagina itself, in a state of lower resistance, or be the consequence of uncured acute vaginitis.

Vaginitis can also be caused by specific infectious agents such as the IBR-IPV virus (infectious pustular vulvo-vaginitis) and *Campylobacter fetus*, which produces enzootic infertility and abortions. Secondary vaginitis is usually the product of the extension of inflammatory processes coming from the cervix or uterus.

General symptoms

Externally, a greyish yellow muco-purulent discharge can be observed in cows when lying down. Sometimes the exudates adhere to the hairs on the lower commissure of the vulva, tail, and buttocks.

Vaginoscopy shows congested, edematous mucosal walls, with collections of exudates on their floor. The more severe the inflammation, the redder and more edematous the mucosa will appear. In these cases, inserting the speculum is difficult.

Diagnosis

Subacute primary vaginitis caused by nonspecific infectious agents is recognized by occurring sporadically in the herd, in cows with a history of retained placentas, acute or subacute metritis. It is important to verify symptoms of inflammation of the vaginal mucosa and cervix, through a meticulous examination with a leaflet speculum.

We have previously said that the simple finding of mucopurulent or purulent secretions in the vagina is not a pathognomonic sign of inflammation. If the cervico-vaginal mucosa is intact and the uterus is healthy, vaginal inflammation must be ruled out.

Subacute primary vaginitis caused by specific infectious agents is recognized as having an enzootic or epizootic contagious nature, that is, it affects a high percentage of animals in the herd and territory. In addition, it is accompanied by concomitant symptoms from other organs. For example, the IBR virus causes infectious pustular vulvovaginitis and rhinotracheitis in cows and balanoposthitis in bulls.

In *Campylobacter fetus* infection, mild vaginal inflammation with exudative discharge may occur, in which the germs can be isolated from the first nine days. But the diagnosis of this venereal disease should be based on temporary collective infertility and early or late abortions, with complications of placental retention.

Treatment

Vaginitis should be treated according to the causes that produce it. Nonspecific ones generally heal on their own. If they are associated with inflammation of the cervix or uterus, it is enough to treat the primary processes. It is not advisable to repeatedly examine inflamed vaginas with a speculum, as the speculum can aggravate the lesions and produce continuous tenesmus. It is best to infuse into the vagina, with a flexible rubber catheter, 100-200 ml of an oily solution or suspension of a broad-spectrum, non-irritating antibiotic. Repeat the dose for three days. Nitrofurazone or solutions such as lugol should not be used due to their irritating effect, much less the intravaginal introduction of candelillas or boluses of sulfonamides or antibiotics. The latter act as foreign bodies and the animals reacts with intense tenesmus to try to expel them. According to experience, *"it is better not to treat than to treat poorly."*

The suspicion of specific vaginitis must be immediately reported to the official Epizootiology authorities, so that the appropriate measures can be taken for its diagnosis, since it may be an important epizootic disease for the country.

Vulvitis and vulvar craurosis

Inflammation of the vulva is rare and when it appears it is associated with trauma that occurred during parturitium. Excessive traction of large calves during birth can cause serious wounds and tears in the vulva, which when healed prevents the labia from coapting properly, facilitating the entry of air or urine into the vagina. This lack of tone and contractile capacity of the vulvar lips is known as vulvar craurosis. The only treatment for this condition is surgical plasty (vulvoplasty), which is a laborious operation and difficult to do successfully under field conditions.

Chapter 7

Abortion and its causes

Content:
Abortion and its types. Analysis of the causes of abortions and the way to deal with them. Measures in the event of serious biological damage.

Introduction

The interruption of pregnancy in bovine herds is a relatively frequent phenomenon and can cause non-compliance with reproductive programs and economic losses. Due to its variety and forms, determining the causes of abortions often becomes a problem. There are several reasons to explain this statement.

Frequently the cause of the abortion occurs weeks or months before it occurs, which makes its diagnosis difficult. Fetuses are retained in the uterus hours and days before being expelled. During that time, they decompose by autolysis, and it is not possible to specify the injuries that occurred in the different organs. Fetal membranes are easily contaminated, making it difficult to establish the primary agent. The toxic agents responsible for abortions often cannot be detected.

Some systemic diseases in the mother can cause abortions even when the reproductive organs are not affected. Many man-made causes of abortion are difficult to recognize.

Abortion and its types

Abortion in cows is defined as fetal death and expulsion between days 45 and 265 of pregnancy. A percentage of 5 % is considered normal.

Two types are known: the one induced by man and the spontaneous or natural one, which is produced by numerous causes (See Table 7-1). The death of the fetus is caused by the direct action of the agent on its organs or indirectly by affecting the fetal or maternal placenta.

Fetal death can occur at an early stage and go unnoticed. If death occurs when the fetus has reached a certain development, three things can happen:

1. The expulsion of the fetus together with its envelopes.
2. Suffer dehydration, called fetal mummification.
3. Suffer liquefaction due to autolytic action, known as fetal maceration.

Although in almost all countries there is systematic control against emerging infectious diseases, it may happen that sanitary gaps occur that allow the penetration of infectious agents into the herd or the reappearance of some that were believed to be controlled. For this reason, it is advisable for the practical veterinarian to be aware of the forms of action in the event of a number of abortions beyond what is considered acceptable in a herd.

Table 7-1 Causes of pregnancy terminations

Non-infectious causes	Infectious causes	
	Viral	
Genetic aberrations	**Desease**	**Agent**
Chromosomal abnormalities	Rinotraqueitis (IBR)	Herpes virus Bovinoi-1
Teratogenic agents		
Nutritional	**Bacterial**	**Agent**
Poisoning toxic plants	Brucelosis	*Brucella abortus*
Nitrate poisoning	Campiiobacteriosis	*Campylobacter fetus*
Vitamin A deficiency	Leptospirosis	*Leptospira pomona*
	Anaplasmosis	*Anaplasma bovis*
Stressors agent	**Protozoan**	**Agent**
Poor handling, racing, bathing	Trichomoniasis	*Trichomonas fetus*
Overheating, heat stroke	Toxoplasmosis	*Toxoplasma gondi*
	Babesiosis	*Babesia bigemina*
Miscellany	**Fungal**	**Agent**
Multiple gestation	Aspergilosis	*Aspergillus spp*
Improper inseminations	Mucormicosis	*Rhizopus, Mucor*
Dehydration		
Transportation, falls		

To do this, you can use the calculation of the percentage of abortions in the herd. This is obtained by dividing the number of abortions that occurred in the period under analysis by the number of cows diagnosed as pregnant, multiplying the resulting result by one hundred.

A recognized abortion rate of 5 % is considered an acceptable loss of pregnancy for a herd over a period of one year. When this index exceeds 10 % there are reasons to worry and the causes that produce it must be sought.

Clinical history of the herd

To direct the steps towards a diagnosis of the causes of abortions, it is necessary to have the following data available:

1- General data of the herd. Location, number of animals.

2- Analysis of reproductive fitness.

Percentage of fertility, gestation, interval between births, percentage of abortions, percentage of retained placenta, percentage of metritis, vaccination program, origin of livestock and their replacements.

Individual clinical history

The data of the cows that interrupted their pregnancy will be very useful, which is why it is necessary to carry individual cards per cow.

These data are:

1. Name and number of the cow. Origin. Age. Number of births, services per conception, number of abortions detected, age of abortion or calf born.
2. Data corresponding to the clinical examination carried out.
3. Detected reproductive diseases: retained placenta, endometritis, metritis.
4. Other clinical data of interest.

Necropsy of fetus

Fetuses and newborn animals are checked similarly to other animals. If possible, the entire fetus, plus the placenta, should be sent to the laboratory as soon as possible.

They will be routinely reviewed:

1. Placenta. Describe its appearance and condition and any macroscopic lesions it presents.

2. The general conditions of the fetus will be reviewed; freshness, degree of autolysis, depigmentation, etc.

3. The thoracic cavity will be examined, from which a portion of the lung and heart will be taken for histopathology (10 % formalin) and another portion of the lung for bacteriology (sterile bottle), which must be kept refrigerated if there are conditions for it.

4. A sample of pericardial fluid or body fluids will be taken (with a syringe), kept refrigerated, and sent to the laboratory for serological testing.

5. The abdominal cavity will be examined, from which portions of the liver, adrenal gland, spleen, and kidney will be taken for histopathology, and liver, kidney and spleen for bacteriology.

6. Stomach contents (1 to 3 ml with a sterile syringe aseptically) will be extracted for microscopic examination and bacteriological isolation. It can be sent in the same syringe, kept under refrigerated conditions, to the laboratory.

Serology

Due to the very nature of the problem, it is common for abortion to be detected several hours or days after its occurrence, so the fetus and placentas may be in an advanced state of autolysis or putrefaction, making them unusable for diagnosis.

For the determination of serum antibodies in the mother, it is necessary to collect blood serum:

1. Take the blood sample in a clean test tube, without anticoagulant.

2. Leave at room temperature for a few hours (do not refrigerate) so that the whey separates.

3. Preferably centrifuge to separate the serum.

4. The whey can be kept refrigerated or frozen.

It is very important to take paired samples (one sample around the abortion and a second 2 to 3 weeks after the first) from the aborted cow, as well as from cows contemporaneous with it (cows from the same pen that have not aborted).

A single sampling is not useful, since it is necessary to study how the antibodies behave from one sampling to the next and between aborted and non-aborted animals in order to establish a possible diagnosis.

Analysis of causes of abortions and their confrontation

Table 7-1 shows the causes of pregnancy interruptions that have the most impact on our herds. Contrary to what one might think, non-infectious causes are the most common. For this reason, when an abortion appears, the best thing to do is go from the simple to the complex. That is, first look at the possible causes provoked by man in his interaction with animals. A characteristic of this type of abortion is its sporadic appearance.

It is important not to include misdiagnoses of pregnancy as abortions, which frequently occur. The health status of pregnant females, their nutritional level, and the management they receive must be checked, including protection against excessive solar irradiation, torrential and continuous rains, etc.

Abortions caused by infectious agents are more dangerous, but less frequent. When they appear, they affect a relatively high number of the females that make up the herd. Among the health gaps that can cause the spread or contagion of infectious diseases, we have the existence of animals of different species living with cows, the incorporation of new animals into the herd without having health certification, the spread of infection by birds. scavengers, stagnant water, etc.

Below is a summarized clinical-epizootiological table of the abortive infectious diseases that are most frequently diagnosed in tropical regions.

Most frequent abortive infectious diseases in the tropics:

Infectious bovine rhinotracheitis

Bovine Herpesvirus-1 causes infectious pustular vulvo-vaginitis. Genital infections can be mild or severe and cause infertility or abortions.

Abortions can occur at any time during pregnancy, but those that occur during the second half are more common. Exposure to BHV-1 of a susceptible herd can cause a spate of abortions, which can reach 25-60% of their pregnant cows.

The infected fetus dies some time before its expulsion, so it generally presents autolytic lesions, and the placenta is frequently retained.

No major changes occur in the fetus, except for the presence of a serohemorrhagic fluid in the cavities and in the fetal body. Signs that help with the diagnosis include foci of necrosis in the liver, spleen, lungs and kidneys.

Brucellosis

Brucella abortus penetrate, via the lymphatic vessels into the maternal-fetal placenta and produce a fibrino-purulent inflammation that leads to the death of the fetus or its weakening and early expulsion.

Infection in cows occurs through amniotic fluid, through the fetus and through lochia, after abortions or premature births. Abortions occur in primiparous females; those who had aborted are immunized and do not abort again.

Clinical symptoms consist of sudden signs of parturition (udder filling), with muco-purulent or muco-bloody vaginal discharge, without odor, and subsequent expulsion of the fetus in the 6th to 8th month of pregnancy.

There is frequently retained placenta affected by yellow gelatinous infiltration, with fibrin and pus. Premature calves that are born alive are weak and die within a few days.

Leptospirosis

Rarely and only in certain areas, sporadic abortion occurs due to infection with leptospires (*Sp. pomona*), in the 7th to 8th month of pregnancy.

Campylobacteriosis

It is a venereal-type infectious disease that causes infertility, embryonic mortality, and abortions between four and seven months of pregnancy. The causative agent is *Campylobacter fetus*, which is a highly mobile *Gram-negative spirillum*. It is in the vagina and uterus, without causing obvious lesions. But in the pregnant animal it moves towards the cotyledons of the gravid uterus, causing them to hemorrhage. The aborted fetus presents a subcutaneous gelatinous edema, and the pleural and pericardial cavity are filled with an abundant fibrino-bloody exudate. The liver increases in size, with necrotic islets and the kidney appears with the capsule separated from the parenchyma by a dense and hemorrhagic fluid.

Trichomoniasis

Tritrichomonas fetus is in the vagina and uterus; it is abundant in the pus of pyometra and in the leucorrheic secretions that accompany abortion. In the fetus they are in the maw, in the cavities and in the connective tissue of the fetus. The disease manifests itself with infertility, abortions and pyometra.

Abortion can be early and complete, that is, the fetus is expelled wrapped with its offspring. It occurs during the first half of pregnancy. Pus is a yellowish-white, lumpy liquid with no distinct odor.

Fetal death may occur, without expulsion, due to the cervix remaining closed. In the absence of bacterial contamination, the dead fetus disintegrates or macerates due to the action of its own enzymes, giving rise to a particular type of chronic endometritis called trichomonas pyometra.

This pyometra differs from the bacterial one by having a lumpy appearance, like that of rice soup, and containing remains of hair and bones.

The diagnosis is best made by testing for live trichomonas in a drop of amniotic fluid or uterine secretions, placed on a slide to be observed at low magnification. Later the discovery of trichomonas in vaginal mucus is uncertain.

As this is a disease transmissible through intercourse, the practical veterinarian must attach great importance to the diagnosis of the affected bull. The best way is to wash the foreskin with 50-80 ml of sterile physiological solution. During washing, an assistant should vigorously massage the foreskin so that the liquid moves throughout the cavity. Once the washing liquid is collected, through a catheter, it is centrifuged, and a drop of the sediment is taken to observe it under a microscope at low magnification.

Anaplasmosis and *Babesiosis* can occasionally cause abortions in *Bos taurus* females of dairy breeds that are not protected against the vectors that transmit them. Zebu females and *Bos taurus* x zebu crossbreeds are naturally resistant to these tropical diseases.

Toxoplasmosis, Aspergillosis and *Mucormycosis* have not been an important cause of abortions in the semi-extensive and extensive breeding conditions of the tropics.

There are other infectious agents capable of causing abortions and reproductive disorders in livestock, but their presence in several tropical countries has not been recognized.

Considering the danger posed by the introduction of exotic diseases, there must be some national emergency plans for the diagnosis and evaluation of biological risk threats, anti-epizootic protection plans and anti-epizootic defense plans. The latter is based on a special technical-administrative organization, designed to act quickly and efficiently in the liquidation of a health emergency.

Action plan in the event of serious biological damage

The action plan must be conceived, known, and practiced by the veterinary staff who have the responsibility of caring for the animals and appear at the place where the first suspicion exists, in such a way that the first cases are not eliminated, clinical observations are carried out. epizootiological and the collection and conservation of the essential samples for a rapid laboratory diagnosis are carried out.

Actions in case of suspicion

The veterinarian will confine the sick animals and will not perform a necropsy until the arrival of the diagnostic group. He will immediately establish the quarantine and notify his immediate superior.

At the breeding site, the veterinarian will ensure the establishment of the counterepizootic measures provided for in the action plan and will deliver to the diagnostic group all the information collected in the general clinical history of the herd and in the individual clinical records, including the observed findings. in abortions and in second births.

Chapter 8

Congenital anomalies

Content:
Introduction. Ovarian hypoplasia. Disease of white heifers. Hermaphroditism. Free-Martinism

---

Introduction

Congenital anomalies of the reproductive tract are defects of structure or function present at birth. They can be lethal or sublethal or compatible with life and have an aesthetic effect that decreases the economic value of the animal. Some anomalies are due to recessive genes and are considered hereditary diseases that, from a zootechnical point of view, are very dangerous, others, although they affect the development of the Müllerian ducts, do not have a genetic origin.

Among the hereditary congenital anomalies compatible with life and affecting reproductive functions, ovarian hypoplasia and white heifer disease have been the most common. The most well-known non-hereditary congenital anomaly is hermaphroditism, which has a low incidence.

Ovarian hypoplasia

In general, pathologists define hypoplasia as a failure of cells, tissues or organs to acquire a mature size. It differs from atrophy in that the atrophic cells have reached their adult size before returning to a diminished form. In particular, ovarian hypoplasia is an alteration in the development of the cortex where the primordial follicles are located. It is produced by a recessive gene of incomplete penetrance that affects the female and the male equally.

Depending on the extent of the lesions, hypoplasia can be complete or partial. In complete hypoplasia, the ovaries, of extremely small volume, do not contain any primordial follicles; In the partial, the ovaries carry some primordial follicles that emit fertilizable ovules.

Hypoplastic ovaries have a reduced volume and their main morphological characteristic consists of the reduction in the number of primordial follicles. However, the ovary retains its general structure: the cortical and medullary layers are present and the *rete ovarii* has a normal appearance. The main alteration is found in the germinal epithelium and the severity of the lesion is parallel to the reduction in the number of follicles. In cases of unilateral ovarian hypoplasia, the most affected ovary is almost always the left one. The tubular portion of the genital apparatus is normal, but insufficiently developed.

The histological study of heifers that present bilateral ovarian hypoplasia always demonstrates little estrogenic activity.

Symptoms

Complete hypoplasia can be bilateral or unilateral. If it is bilateral, the ovaries, uterus and vulva of the heifer are poorly developed. The udder is small and lacking elasticity, with rudimentary teats, with a hard and compact consistency. The affected female looks like a castrated steer since her ovaries do not function.

In *complete unilateral hypoplasia*, the affected ovary is almost always the left one, which appears as a simple bulge, of a hard consistency, in the broad ligament and does not exceed the volume of a pea. The rest of the genital apparatus does not show obvious changes, but the animal has low fertility and requires several services to become fertilized. Jealousy is not very expressive and the interpartum intervals are prolonged.

In *partial hypoplasia*, lesions can occur in both ovaries, which have a reduced volume. The other symptoms are like those of complete unilateral hypoplasia already described.

Diagnosis

I must say that, due to its low incidence, ovarian hypoplasia as a cause of sterility in Cuban livestock is of little importance. However, it has happened and may continue to happen that interpretive errors are made when performing rectal examination of the ovaries of Bos indicus heifers and cows and their crosses with Bos taurus, which can have very small and small normal ovaries, especially the left one. See Chapter 4.

Complete and *bilateral ovarian hypoplasia* differs from the others in that it can be recognized externally by the vulvar and mammary underdevelopment of the heifer that suffers from it; They are also sterile, so, from a zootechnical point of view, they do not represent any danger.

In *complete unilateral hypoplasia* the most indicative sign is the reduction in the volume of one of the ovaries, up to two or three times smaller than the healthy one.

This comparative state of size between ovaries is important since, in cases of heifers that normally have small ovaries, the difference between the left and right ovaries almost never exceeds 5 mm. In this type of hypoplasia, there are no changes in the external habit of the animal, but it may show some delay in the onset of puberty and have a low fertility potential, which is abnormal in a heifer.

In *partial hypoplasia*, the diagnosis is difficult since there are no distinctive clinical symptoms and this is the most dangerous thing because the animal is fertile and transmits the disease to its children. If the offspring is male, testicular hypoplasia occurs and in this case the male becomes the spreader of the disease. Only by identifying and locating the parents of hypoplastic children, is it possible to break the chain of transmission of this hereditary disease.

Treatment

Hereditary diseases have no treatment. Any female diagnosed as hypoplastic must be eliminated from the herd, as should her parents wherever they are found.

White heifer disease

This hereditary disease gets its name from having been described for the first time in white-coated Shorthorn females in Belgium, although it can appear, more rarely, in heifers of other European breeds. The anomaly is characterized by modifications in the development and differentiation of the organs derived from the Müllerian ducts (uterus, tubes and vagina), associated or not with anomalies of the hymen, or the presence of organs derived from the Wolffian ducts.

Etiology

Heredity plays a decisive role since too close consanguinity contributes to revealing the disease. It is produced by an autosomal recessive gene, whose action is associated or favored by the presence of the white factor, but this does not explain its appearance in other dark-coat breeds.

Lesions

Hymen anomalies are the most common. The hymen can be completely imperforate, perforated in the center or found in the form of medial or lateral flanges. In some subjects the constriction of the hymenal ring is so strong that it prevents the introduction of the speculum. When the hymen is completely imperforate, it causes the formation of a cystic sac that contains variable amounts of fluid that makes urination and defecation difficult.

The vagina may be absent, imperforate, shortened or closed.

Uterine anomalies consist of segmental aplasia or cystic dilation. Generally, the lesions are bilateral, but they can affect only one horn and in that case fertilization is possible.

Other times the horns are rudimentary, clearly hypoplastic, or reduced to fibrous bands of variable length. The body and cervix of the uterus are sometimes absent or replaced by a fibrous flange of varying thickness.

The ovaries are always present and functional, therefore, the female with this disease can be in heat normally.

Symptoms

Fertility varies depending on the degree and importance of the abnormalities. The mere existence of the hymenal membrane is not an obstacle to fertilization. Estrus is almost always regular in duration and intensity. The vulva and clitoris are almost always well-developed unlike the *Freemartin*, in which there is a subnormal external genitourinary opening and a protruding clitoris. The white heifer appears externally as a normal female, unlike the *Freemartin* which has the appearance of a neutral, intersexual type.

Incidence and prognosis

In my experience of more than four decades of teaching and clinical work, I could not find any case of this anomaly. However, it is always advisable to know its existence and be alert to its eventual appearance. Furthermore, the description of its injuries can serve to differentiate it from other similar disorders.

Since subjects who only present persistence of the hymen are fertile, the danger of spread makes the prognosis of this hereditary disease extremely serious, from a gynecological and zootechnical point of view. If the disease is identified within a family, all carriers, including parents, must be eliminated.

Hermaphroditism

It is an anomaly characterized by the existence, in the same individual, of genital organs belonging to both sexes. Anomalies may occur on the copulatory organs (external hermaphroditism), the genital tract (tubular hermaphroditism) or the genital glands (glandular hermaphroditism). This anomaly is found in different species, particularly pigs and goats.

Pseudohermaphrodites are those animals that have the internal reproductive organs of one sex, but their external appearance is that of the other sex.

In cattle a particular type of male pseudo-hermaphroditism called *Freemartin* occurs with low frequency.

Freemartinism

The *Freemartin* is a sterile heifer born from a twin birth with a male. This intersex occurs in 90 % of twins of both sexes, the remaining 10 % are normal.

Pathogenesis and lesions

The existence of freemartinism is known only in cattle and seems to be related to the fusion of the chorion and the allantois during twin pregnancies in which fetuses of both sexes develop. The vascular anastomosis between the two fetuses is followed by the passage of embryonic erythrocyte cells that establish themselves in the hematopoietic tissues of the host, where they remain in a functional state throughout the course of life.

That is, erythro-mosaicism occurs in which each twin has a mixture of antigenically different erythrocytes.

Symptoms

An intermediate type *Freemartin* heifer can be presented, in which the animal has rudimentary ovaries, a small uterus, an imperforate vagina, an infantile vulva, with a normal clitoris and the presence of small epididymis or vas deferens.

In the asexual *Freemartin* type, the heifer has rudimentary ovaries and breasts, absence or very little development of the uterus, a subnormal genitourinary opening, and a long and protruding clitoris. In some cases, small testicles can be palpated below the udder and the animal looks and behaves like a male (rough skin, protruding chest, jumping on other females).

Diagnosis

It will be based on the external appearance of the animal, on the abnormal development of the clitoris, on the absence or insufficiency of the development of the internal genital organs and the udder.

Since a twin pregnancy of different sexes is essential for a *Freemartin* to be produced, its spontaneous appearance in herds is very low. However, when treatments with the PMSG hormone are used to induce heat in anestric females, the probabilities of the appearance of this intersex increase since PMSG, even in low doses, can produce superovulation. Therefore, this factor must be considered.

Bibliography

Acosta Clarisa M., Jiménez Celia R. (1987): Influencias del sistema de explotación y manejo sobre el comportamiento reproductivo de vacas mestizas ¾ B.S x ¼ C y ¾ HS Rojo x ¼ C. en la provincia de Villa Clara. Orientador Científico Luis O. Alba. Trabajo de Diploma. Facultad Ciencia Animal, Universidad Central de las Villas.

Alabart, J., Folch y E. Calvo (1985): La inmunización contra esteroides como método para aumentar la prolíficidad en el ganado ovino. ITEA Producción Animal Extra (5):317-318.

Alba, L. O. y Armengol J. A. (1976): Influencias de las épocas del año, métodos de crianza y sistemas de explotación, sobre el comportamiento reproductivo de vacas mestizas Brown Swiss x cebú y Holstein x cebú en algunas unidades de la Provincia de Villa Clara. II Congreso Nacional de Medicina Veterinaria, pp 25, noviembre. La Habana.

Alba L. O., Rodríguez G., Gómez A. Silveira E. (2006): Tamaño y forma de los ovarios y de la cerviz en novillas y vacas del cruzamiento absorbente Holstein x Cebú. REDVET VI I (03):10-16.

Alba, L.O. (1987): Nuevos aspectos sobre la significación diagnóstica de las secreciones cérvico-vaginales mucopurulentas y purulentas en las hembras vacunas. III Seminario Internacional de Medicina Veterinaria. CENSA, La Habana.

Alba, L.O., Koutinhoin B. y Torres, L. (1999): La disfunción del cuerpo lúteo como posible causa de repeticiones de servicios de la vaca Holstein en la región central de Cuba. Archivos de Reproducción Animal, ARA, 8:40-45.

Alba L.O., Guadalupe Hernández, Silveira E., Cruz E., Maroto L.O. (2005): Hallazgo de una leucorrea vaginal de carácter no inflamatoria en hembras bovinas. I. Examen macroscópico y microscópico. REDVET 6(10):10-18.

Alba L.O., Segredo E., Silveira E., Cruz E., Maroto L.O. (2005): Hallazgo de una leucorrea vaginal de carácter no inflamatoria en hembras bovinas. II. Pesquisa microbiológica vaginal y uterino REDVET 6(10):18-26.

Alba L.O., Armas J., Fernández A., Rojas Delfa (1977): Flora bacteriológica y uterina de vacas clínicamente sanas en diferentes períodos del ciclo estral. VI Reunión Asociación Latinoamericana de Producción Animal, La Habana.

Alba L.O., Segredo E. (2005): Hallazgo de una leucorrea vaginal de carácter no inflamatoria en hembras bovinas. II. Pesquisaje microbiológico vaginal y uterino. Revista Electrónica de Veterinaria REDVET 6(10):19-24.

Alba L.O., Casañas H., Silveira E. (2005): Hallazgo de una leucorrea vaginal de carácter no inflamatoria en hembras bovinas. III. Características clínicas y fertilidad. Revista Electrónica de Veterinaria REDVET 6(10):1-9.

Alba L.O. y Silveira E. (2006): La leucorrea vaginal bovina de carácter no inflamatorio y su significación clínica. REDVET 7(10):1-9.

Alcántara J. M. (2000): Comportamiento reproductivo histórico y actual de un rebaño de hembras. Siboney de Cuba perteneciente a la Empresa Pecuaria V Congreso Venegas. Orientador Científico Luis O. Alba. Trabajo de Curso. Sede Universitaria, Sancti Spíritus.

Alvarez, R. Carvalho B. Silva A. Perone C. Rivela C and Olivera F. (1997): Endocrine profiles and ovulation rate in cows superovulated with FSH following passive inmunization against steroid free-bovine follicular fluid. Therionology 47(1):164.

Ayala, L., Pesantez, José., Rodas, E., Méndez María Silvana, Soria, M., et al (2017): Tamaño del folículo ovulatorio, cuerpo lúteo y progesterona sanguínea en vaquillas receptoras de embriones de tres razas en pastoreo en Ecuador. Rev. prod. anim., 29 (2), 65-72.

Barr, B.C. and Anderson M. (1993): Infections diseases causing bovine and fetal loss. Vet. Clin North Am. Food. Anim. Pract. 9:343.

Barr, B.C. and Bon Durant R. (1997): Viral Diseases of the fetus. En: R.S. Youngquist ed. Current Therapy in Large Animal, Theriogenology. W.B. Saunders company, Philadelphia.

BonDurant RH. (1999): Inflammation in the bovine female reproductive tract. J Anim Sci Suppl. 2:101-110.

Boyd J. S., Omran S.N., Ayliffe T.R. (1998): Use of a high frequency transducer with real time B-mode ultrasound scanning to identify early pregnancy in cows. Vet. Rec. 121:8-11.

Brito, R., Tobada P., Pedroso R., Preval B., Segui J. (1999): Inducción y sincronización de celo en el ganado cebú, en sistema de manejo extensivo. Archivos de Reproducción Animal, ARA, 8:6-16.

Brito, R. (1999): Fisiología de la Reproducción Animal con Elementos de Biotecnología. Primera Ed. Ed. Félix Varela, La Habana, Tema 2, p 61.

Brito, R y Preval, B. (1989): Inducción del parto en la vaca. Rev, Cub Cienc. Vet., 20(4):219-222.

Brown L., Odde K, King M, LeFever D, Neubauer C. (1988): Comparison of MGA-$PGF_{2\alpha}$ to Syncro-Mate B for estrous synchronization in beef heifers. Theriogenology, 30:1.

Butt B., Senger P., Widders P. (1991): Neutrophil migration into the bovine uterine lumen following intrauterine inoculation with killed *Haemophilus somnus*. J Reprod Fert. 93:341-345.

Caccia M, Bo G. A. (1998): Synchronizing follicle wave emergence following treatment of CIDR-B implanted beef cows with estradiol benzoate and progesterone. Theriogenology, 49(1):341, abstr.

Caccia M, Ungerfield R, Goñi C, Bo G. (1996): Efecto de la dosis y vía de administración del benzoato de estradiol en vacas con CIDR-B. 2do Simposio Internacional de Reproducción Animal, 249. Córdoba, Argentina.

Campbell B, McNeilly A, Picton H, Baird D. (1990): The effect of a potent gonadotrophin-releasing hormone antagonist on ovarian secretion of oestradiol, inhibin and androstenedione and the concentration of LH and FSH during the follicular phase of the oestrus cycle. J. Endocrinol, 126:377-384.

Chacin M, Hansen P., Drost M. (1990): Effects of the stage of estrous cycle and steroid treatment on uterine immunoglobulin content and polymorphonuclear leukocytes in cattle. Theriogenology. 4:1169–1184.

Crowe, M., Enright W. Swift, P and Roche J. (1995): Growth and estrus behavior of heifers actively immunized against PGFα. J. Anim. Sci. 73(2):345-352.

Crowe, M.; Roche J. and, Enright W. (1996): Administration of PGF2α to heifers with pesistent corpora lutea following PGF2α immunization: oestrus and ovarian responses. Anim. Reprod. Sci. 44(2):71-78.

Cruz, R.; Soto, E.; Rincón, E.; González, C. y Villamediana, P. (1998): Evaluación ultrasonográfica de la dinámica folicular en vacas y en novillas mestizas. Revista Científica FCV-LUZ, 8 (1), 14- 24.

Custer E, Beal W, Hall S, Meadows A, Berardinelli J y Adair R. (1994): Effect of melengestrol acetate (MGA) or progesterone-releasing intravaginal devices (PRID) of follicular development, estradiol-17β and progesterone concentrations luteinizing hormone release during an artificially lengthened bovine estrous cycle. J Anim Sci, 72:1282-1289.

Dekeiser, J. (1986): Bovine genital campylobacteriosis. In Current Therapy in Theriogenology Ed. Morrow, D. 2 W. Saunders, Company, Philadelphia.

Dimoso, Z. J. (1984.): Estudio cualitativo y cuantitativo de la flora bacteriológica de las secreciones cervico-uterinas de vacas clínicamente sanas. Orientador Científico Agustín Fernández. Trabajo de Diploma. Facultad de Ciencia Animal. Universidad Central de las Villas. Santa Clara, 1984.

Elliott, L., McMahon, K.J., Gier, H. & Marion, G.B. (1968): Uterus of the cow after parturition: bacterial content. Am. J. Vet. Res. 29, 77-81.

Fenner, F.J. Gibbs E.P., Murphy, F.A. et al. (1993): Herpesviridae. in Veterinary Virology. Academy Press, New York.

Fernández, A., Villavicencio, L., Peláez. R., Silveira, E. y García, Paulina (1984): Estudio cualitativo y cuantitativo de la microflora de secreciones cervicouterinas en vacas con repetición de celo. Rev. Cub. Reprod. Anim. 10(2): 83- 93.

García J. L. (1993): Comportamiento reproductivo comparativo en las vacas. Holstein de Dos Ríos antes y después de la supresión de alimentos concentrados a la ración. Orientador Científico Luis O. Alba. Trabajo de Diploma, Facultad de Ciencias Agropecuaria. Filial Universitaria. José Martí, de Sancti Spíritus.

García Paulina, Martínez Elena, Peraza Nayda, González J. (1990): Estudio comparativo del comportamiento de la microflora cérvico-vaginal en hembras recién paridas clínicamente sanas, con endometritis y repitentes de la raza Holstein y sus cruces. Rev Cub Reprod Anim 18(2):25-35.

Garverick H.A. (1997): Ovarian follicular cysts in dairy cows. J Dairy Sci80:995-1004.

Gil, A; Agüero F. y Faure R. (1997): Diagnóstico precoz de la no gestación en bovinos con benzoato de estradiol. XII Jornada Científica CIMA. La Habana, 3-6 junio, p 5.

Ginther O. J. (1995): Ultrasonic imaging and animal reproduction: Fundamentals, Book 1. Ginther Ed. Madison, Wisconsin.

Gong J, Bramley T., Webb R. (1991): The effect of recombinant bovine somatotropin on ovarian function in heifers: follicular populations and peripheral hormones. Biol Reprod, 45:941-949.

Gonzalez A, Lussier J, Carruthers T, Murphy B, Mapletoft R. (1990): Superovulation of beef heifers with Folltropin-V: a new FSH preparation containing reduced LH activity. Theriogenology, 33:519.

Holy, L. (1987): Biología de la Reproducción Bovina. 2da Ed. Editorial Científico-Técnico, La Habana, Cap. III, pp 3 y 22.

Hussain A., Daniel R., O'Boyle D. (1990): Postpartum uterine flora following normal and abnormal puerperium in cows. Theriogenology 34:291-302.

Kaneko H, Nakanishi Y, Akag S, Ami K, Taya K, Watanabe G, Sasamoto S, Hasegawa Y. (1995): Immunoneutralization of inhibin and estradiol during the follicular phase of the estrous cycle in cows. Biol Reprod, 53:931-939.

Kesler D., Favero R. (1995): Estrus synchronization in beef females with norgestomet and estradiol valerate. Part 1: Mechanism of action. Agri-Practice, 16 (10).

Kimsey, P.B. (1986): Bovine trichomoniasis. En: Morrow, D. A. ed. Current Therapy in Theriogenology 2:275- 279.

Kouba, V. (2003): Epizootiology. Principles and Methods. Institute of Tropical and Subtropical Agriculture. Czech University of Agriculture Prague. Electronic book, pp 199.

Lennite, V., L. Delaby, J. Ihimonier, R. Dufour and M Terqui (1993): Effect of passive immunization against testosterone on reproductive hormone secretion and ovarian function in dairy cows and pubertal beef heifers. *Theriogenology.* 39(2):507-526.

Lliteras, Emilia., Noelia González, R. Pedroso, M. Bravo, N. Felipe (1995): Efecto de la inmunización activa contra esteroides sobre la aparición de la actividad cíclica en borregas Pelibuey. X Forum de Ciencia y Técnica del CIMA. La Habana.

MacDonald, L. E. (1991): Endocrinología Veterinaria y Reproducción. 4ta Ed. Nueva Editorial Interamericana Mc. Graw-Hill, México.

MacMillan KL, Peterson AJ. (1993): A new intravaginal progesterone releasing device for cattle (CIDR-B) for oestrous synchronisation, increasing pregnancy rates and the treatment of post-partum anoestrus. Anim Reprod Sci, 26: 25-40.

MacMillan KL, Thatcher WW. (1991): Effects of an agonist of gonadotropin releasing hormone on ovarian follicles in cattle. Biol Reprod; 45:883-889.

Martínez G., Solano R., Ricardo E., Alcalá L. y Mika Y. (1985): Análisis del comportamiento reproductivo de un rebaño de hembras cebú. IV. Efecto de algunos factores climáticos sobre el comportamiento reproductivo. Rev. Cub. Reprod. Anim. 11(1):81-98.

Miller, J.M. (1991): The effects of IBR virus infection on reproductive function of cattle. Vet. Med. 86:95.

Nell, T. and Gielsen J. (1995): The development of a monoclonal antibody against PMSG for veterinary application. Livest. Prod. Sci. 42(2-3):223-228.

Newton, G.R., Mortinod, S., Hansen P. et al. (1990): Effect of bovine interferon on acute change in body temperature and serum progesterone concentration in heifers. J. Dairy Sci. 73(3):439-448.

Nicoletti, P. (1993): Brucellocis. En: Howard, J.L. (ed) Current Veterinary Therapy: Food Animal Practice, W.B. Saunders Company, Philadelphia.

O'Farrel, K. (1979): Betamethasone induced calving: A comparison between induced and not induced dairy cows. Calving problems and early viability of the calf. Current Topics in Vet. Med. and Anim. Sci. 4:341-351.

Patterson D., Nieman N., Nelson C., Schillo K, Bullock K, Brophy D, Woods B. (1997): Estrus synchronization with an oral progestogen prior to superovulation of postpartum beef cows. Theriogenology, 48:1025-1033.

Perdigón, F., Alba, L. O. (1988): Características anatómicas de los ovarios de hembras de la raza Santa Gertrudis y algunos aspectos de su comportamiento reproductivo. VI Conferencia de Ciencias Agropecuarias, Universidad Central, Cuba.

Peter, D. (1997): Bovine venereal diseases in: Current Therapy in Large Animal R.S. Yongquist ed. Theriogenology. W.B. Saunders Company, Philadelphia.

Preval B. (2000): Utilización de la lidocaína como base en el tratamiento de la retención placentaria, la metritis puerperal e incremento de la fertilidad. Orientador Científico Roberto Brito. Tesis de doctorado. UNAH, La Habana.

Preval, B. (1995): Utilización de la lidocaína como base, en el tratamiento de la retención placentaria, la metritis puerperal e incremento de la fertilidad. Orientador Científico Roberto Brito. Tesis de Doctorado, UNAH, La Habana.

Ryan, D.P., Frichad J.F., Kopel E. and Godke A. (1993): Comparing early embryo mortality in dairy cows during hot and cool seasons of the year. Theriogenology, 39:719-737.

Solano, R., Martínez G., Iglesias C., Ineida Montes (1979): Efecto de dos tratamientos a base de antibióticos y solución lugol, en vacas anéstricas y repitentes. Rev. Cub. Reprod. Anim. 5:13.

Trowbridge H., Emling F. (1997): Hypersensitivity reactions. En: Inflammation: A Review of the Process. 5th ed.pp 111–127 Quintessence Publishing Co., Inc., Chicago, IL.

Watson E.D (1985): Opsonising ability of bovine uterine secretions during the oestrous cycle. Vet Rec. 117:274–275.

Wira CR, Kaushic C. (1996): Mucosal immunity in the female reproductive tract: effect of sex hormones on immune recognition and responses. En: MucosalVaccines. H Kiyono, PL Ogra, JR McGhee, pp 375–388. Academic Press, San Diego, CA.

Wira C., Rossoll R. (1995): Antigen presenting cells in the female reproductive tract: Influence of estrous cycle on antigen presentation by uterine epithelial and stromal cells. Endocrinology. 136:4526–4534.

Woolums A., Peter A. (1994): Cystic Ovarian Condition in Cattle. Part II. Pathogenesis and treatment. Compendium on continuing. Education for the practicing Veterinarian. 16(9): 1247-1250.

Zerbe H, Schuberth H., Hoedemaker M, Grunert E, Leibold W. (1996): A new model system for endometritis: basic concepts and characterization of phenotypic and functional properties.

Glossary of some terms used in reproduction

Abortion: Expulsion before full term of a conceptus which is incapable of independent life.
Anoestrus: Lack of oestrus behavior. The animal has not cyclic activity on the ovaries.
Body condition: Method of assessment of the degree of fatness and condition of the animal based on estimation of backfat thickness.
Breeding: Any activity assuring the placement of semen into the genital tract of a receptive female by natural or artificial means.
Breeding season: Period of maximal reproductive activity in non-pregnant animals.
Calving interval: Interval between successive parturitions in cattle.
Conception rate: Number of animals pregnant, expressed as a percentage of the total number mated or inseminated.
Conceptus: The product of conception throughout the entire period of gestation.
Embryo: Conceptus during the period of differentiation.
Embryonic mortality: The death or loss of the conceptus during the period between conception and completion of differentiation.
Exogenous hormone: Hormone (natural or synthetic) which is administered to an animal.
Follicle: Fluid-filled ovarian structure contained the oocyte.
Hand mating: Controlled mating usually performed after grouping of oestrus.
Immunization techniques: Modification of reproductive functions through stimulation of antibodies against endogenous hormones by vaccination.

Intersexuality: Presence of gonadal tissue of both sexes in the same individual. Also known as hermaphroditism.
Libido: Sexual drive, specially of males.
Mating: Act of sexual intercourse. In the absence of visual observation, the term is joining.
Non-return rate: Percentage of the animals not seen to return to after service or AI in a defined period after service or AI.
Pheromone: Odoriferous substance given out by one animal that act a signal to another of the same species.
Repeat breeder cow: Cow, without apparent clinical abnormalities, that did not conceive after at least three successive mating or AI.
Retained placenta: Retention of fetal membranes after parturition >24 hours in cattle.
Standing reflex: Reaction on immobility of a female in heat to the stimulus of the male (or the females) which allow mounting.
Teaser bull: Entire or vasectomized bull generally sed to stimulate females, or to facilitate oestrus detection.
Vasectomy: Surgical section of the deferent tubules of the testicles resulting in sterility without affecting libido.
Zebu crossbred: Zebu female product of interracial crossing of *Bos indicus.*

Biographical summary

The author Luis Orlando Alba Gómez, PhD, Full Professor, Expert in Bovine Reproduction. Former Head of the Chair of Animal Reproduction for 50 years at the Central University of L.V. and José Martí in Sancti Spiritus, Cuba. He supervised more than 30 Diploma Theses, 15 Specialization Theses and two PhDs in Veterinary Sciences. He has published 28 articles in magazines and three scientific books.

2

www.ingramcontent.com/pod-product-compliance
Lightning Source LLC
Chambersburg PA
CBHW071829210526
45479CB00001B/53